Self-Assessment Color Review of

Respiratory Medicine

Stephen G. Spiro

BSc, MD, FRCP
Head, Division of Respiratory Medicine
Clinical Director of Medicine
University College London Hospitals, UK

Richard K. Albert

MD
Professor of Medicine
University of Washington
Section Head, Pulmonary and Critical Care Medicine
University of Washington Medical Center
Seattle, WA, USA

David Fielding

FRACP
Honorary Senior Respiratory Registrar
University College London Hospitals, UK

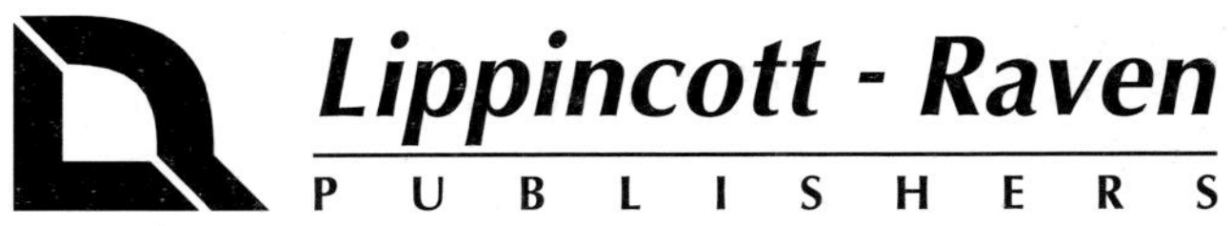

Acknowledgements

For their help in preparing this book we thank Dr Simon Abel (Registrar, Papworth Hospital, Cambridge), Dr J. Bomanji (Department of Nuclear Medicine, University College London Hospitals), Dr Merryl Griffiths (Department of Nuclear Medicine, University College London Hospitals), and Dr Martin Hetzel (Department of Nuclear Medicine, University College London Hospitals).

Published 1997 in North America by:
Lippincott–Raven Publishers,
227 East Washington Square,
Philadelphia, PA 19106–3780
ISBN 0–316–80697–8

Library of Congress Cataloging-in-Publication data applied for.

A CIP catalogue record for this book is available from the British Library.

For full details of all Manson Publishing Ltd titles please write to
Manson Publishing Ltd, 73 Corringham Road, London NW11 7DL, UK.

Design and layout: The Little Round Consultancy
Text editing and proof-reading: William Down and Mary Korndorffer
Colour reproduction: Reed Reprographics, Ipswich, UK
Printed by: Grafos SA, Barcelona, Spain

Preface

Students and practitioners of respiratory medicine are aware that it covers many diverse areas and encompasses about 25% of all general medical problems. The questions and answers in this book aim to present key points on topics across this spectrum of diseases. There are proportionally more problems on the common disorders, including lung cancer, obstructive airways disease and pulmonary infections. Other topics include lung function testing, occupational medicine, sleep medicine, intensive care, interventional techniques, thoracic surgery, pulmonary vascular disease, immunologic disorders, nasal pathology and pulmonary fibrosis. Pulmonary manifestations of systemic disease and human immunodeficiency virus are also covered.

The aim of this book is to increase the reader's understanding of clinically relevant topics by providing explanatory answers; it is more than a book of spot diagnosis questions or a catalogue of rare conditions with interesting radiological featurs which the reader simply knows or does not.

The contributors have extensive experience in their specialized fields and have described situations which reflect actual practice, in so far as is possible. Several have just completed their specialist training and have provided questions that they consider of particular value to those undergoing specialist accreditation. Furthermore, by presenting the questions in pictorial form we hope that the problems become more interesting and the material easier to remember for the reader.

Stephen G. Spiro
University College London Hospitals
London, UK

Richard K. Albert
University of Washington Medical Center
Seattle, USA

David Fielding
University College London Hospitals
London, UK

Contributors

Roger Allen, FCCP, FRACP, PhD
Consultant Respiratory Physician
Clinical Associate Professor
Prince Charles Hospital
Brisbane, Australia

Griffith M. Blackmon, MD
Senior Fellow/Acting Instructor
University of Washington Medical
Center, Seattle, USA

M. Gary Brook, MRCP
Senior Registrar
University College London Hospitals,
London, UK

Feroza Daroowalla, MD
Senior Fellow/Acting Instructor
University of Washington Medical
Center, Seattle, USA

David Fielding, FRACP
Hon. Senior Respiratory Registrar
University College London Hospitals,
London, UK

Rebecca Fox-Dewhurst, MD
Senior Fellow/Acting Instructor
University of Washington Medical
Center, Seattle, USA

Vishesh Kapur, MD
Senior Fellow/Acting Instructor
University of Washington Medical
Center, Seattle, USA

Margaret Krieg, MD
Senior Fellow/Acting Instructor
University of Washington Medical
Center, Seattle, USA

Alan W. Matthews, MD, FRCP
Consultant Physician
Queen Alexandra Hospital, Portsmouth,
UK

Robert F. Miller, MRCP
Senior Lecturer
Honorary Consultant Physician
University College London Hospitals,
London, UK

David R. Park, MD
Senior Fellow/Acting Instructor
University of Washington Medical
Center, Seattle, USA

Wilfred B. Pugsley, FRCS
Consultant Cardiothoracic Surgeon
University College London Hospitals,
London, UK

Stephen G. Spiro, BSc, MD, FRCP
Head, Division of Respiratory Medicine
Clinical Director of Medicine
University College London Hospitals,
London, UK

Eric M. Stern, MD
Associate Professor of Radiology
University of Washington Medical
Center, Seattle, USA

Yoke Khim Tan, M. Med
Visiting Senior Registrar
University College London Hospitals,
London, UK

David F. Treacher, MRCP
Consultant Physician
Director of Intensive Care
St Thomas' Hospital, London, UK

William Walker, FRCP
Consultant Cardiothoracic Surgeon
City Hospital
Edinburgh, UK

Bennet M. Wang, MD
Senior Fellow/Acting Instructor
University of Washington Medical
Center, Seattle, USA

A. Kevin Webb, MRCP
Consultant Chest Physician
Wythenshawe Hospital
Manchester, UK

Mark Woodhead, MRCP
Consultant in General and
Respiratory Medicine
Manchester Royal Infirmary
Manchester, UK

Abbreviations

2D	two-dimensional
ABPA	allergic bronchopulmonary aspergillosis
ACE	angiotensin converting enzyme
ACTH	adrenocorticotrophic hormone
AFB	acid fast bacilli
AHI	apnoea–hypoapnoea index
AIDS	acquired immune dficiency syndrome
ANCA	anti-cytoplasmic antibodies
AP	anterioposterior
ARDS	acute respiratory distress syndrome
BAL	bronchoalveolar lavage
BMT	bone marrow transplant
CF	cystic fibrosis
CFA	cryptogenic fibrosing alveolitis
CMV	cytomegalovirus
CNS	central nervous system
COAD	chronic obstructive airways disease
COPD	chronic obstructive pulmonary disease
CPAP	continuous positive airways pressure
CRP	C-reactive protein
CSF	cerebrospinal fluid
CT	computed tomography
CWP	coal workers' pneumoconiosis
DIC	disseminated intravascular coagulation
DIOS	distal intestinal obstruction syndrome
DL_{CO}	diffusion coefficient for carbon monoxide
DNA	deoxyribonucleic acid
DTPA	diethylenetriamine penta-acetate
ECG	electrocardiogram
EEG	electroencephalogram
EMG	electromyogram
ERV	expiratory reserve volume
ESR	erythrocyte sedimentation rate
ET	endotracheal
FEV	forced expiratory volume
FRC	functional residual capacity
FVC	forced vital capacity
GM-CSF	granulocyte–macrophage colony stimulating factor
HCG	human chorionic gonadotropin
HDI	hexamethylene diisocyanate
HIV	human immunodeficiency virus
HLA	human leukocyte antigen
HP	hypersensitivity pneumonitis
HPOA	hypertrophic pulmonary osteoarthropathy
HRCT	high-resolution computed tomography
ICS	inhaled corticosteroids
IL	interleukin
ILO	International Labour Organization
IPF	idiopathic pulmonary fibrosis
JVP	jugular venous pressure
KS	Kaposi's sarcoma
LEMS	Lambert–Eaton syndrome
LIP	lymphocytic interstitial pneumonitis
LTOT	long-term oxygen therapy
LVF	left ventricular failure
MAC	*Mycobacterium avium-intracellulare* complex
MAP	mean arterial pressure
MDI	(diphenyl) methane diisocyanate
MHC	major histocompatability complex
MRC	Medical Research Council
MRI	magnetic resonance imaging
MSLT	multiple sleep latency testing
MST	morphine sulphate continuous
MVV	maximal voluntary ventilation
NOTT	Nocturnal Oxygen Therapy Trial
OCS	oral corticosteroids

Abbreviations

OLB	open lung biopsy		REM	rapid eye movement (sleep)
OSA	obstructive sleep apnoea		RLS	restless leg syndrome
PA	posterioanterior		RQ	respiratory exchange ratio (quotient)
PAN	polyarteritis nodosa			
PAOP	pulmonary artery occlusion (wedge) pressure		RV	residual volume
			SCLC	small-cell lung cancer
PAP	pulmonary artery pressure		SIADH	syndrome of inappropriate anti-diuretic hormone secretion
PAS	periodic acid–Schiff			
PCP	*Pneumocystis carinii* pneumonitis			
			SLE	systemic lupus erythematosus
PDT	photodynamic therapy		SVCO	superior vena caval obstruction
PE	pulmonary embolism			
PEEP	positive end-expiratory pressure		TDI	toluene diisocyanate
			TGF	transforming growth factor
PEFR	peak expiratory flow rate		TLC	total lung capacity
PIE	pulmonary infiltrates with eosinophilia (syndrome)		TNF	tumour necrosis factor
			TNM	tumour classification system
PIOPED	prospective investigation of pulmonary embolism diagnosis		UAWO	upper airway obstruction
			UPPP	uvulopalatopharyngoplasty
			VATS	video-assisted thoracoscopic surgery
PLMS	periodic limb movement in sleep			
			VA	alveolar volume
PMF	progressive massive fibrosis		VC	vital capacity
PTE	pulmonary thromboembolism		VD	dead space
RAP	right atrial pressure		YAG	yttrium aluminium garnet

Bacterial, fungal and other organism abbreviations

A. fumigatus	*Aspergillus fumigatus*		*M. tuberculosis*	*Mycobacterium tuberculosis*
B. cepacia	*Burkholderia cepacia*			
C. albicans	*Candida albicans*		*Myc. pneumoniae*	*Mycoplasma pneumoniae*
C. burnetti	*Coxiella burnetti*			
C. neoformans	*Cryptococcus neoformans*		*P. carinii*	*Pneumocystis carinii*
			P. aeruginosa	*Pseudomonas aeruginosa*
C. psittaci	*Chlamydia psittaci*			
E. coli	*Escherichia coli*		*P. pseudomallei*	*Pseudomonas pseudomallei*
H. influenza	*Haemophilus influenza*			
			S. haemotibia	*Schistosoma haemotibia*
K. pneumoniae	*Klebsiella pneumoniae*			
L. pneumophila	*Legionella pneumophila*		*S. japonica*	*Schistosoma japonica*
			S. mansoni	*Schistosoma mansoni*
M. avium	*Mycobacterium avium*		*Staph. aureus*	*Staphylococcus aureus*
M. intracellulare	*Mycobacterium intracellulare*			
			Str. pneumoniae	*Streptococcus pneumoniae*
M. kansasii	*Mycobacterium kansasii*		*T. gondii*	*Toxoplasma gondii*

1 This HIV-positive man has developed several new lesions, as that in **1a**.
i. What is the diagnosis?
ii. How and when may the lung be affected by this condition and what is its therapy?

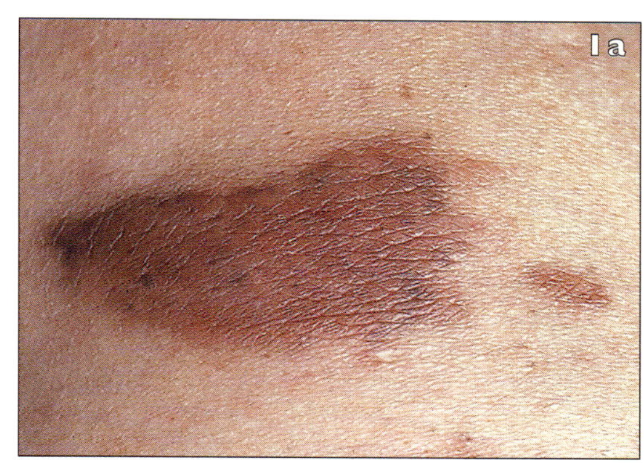

2 **i.** What stain has been employed on this endobronchial biopsy (**2a**, **2b**)?
ii. Is this positive staining specific for this condition?
iii. Are these tumours usually confined to within the bronchial lumen?

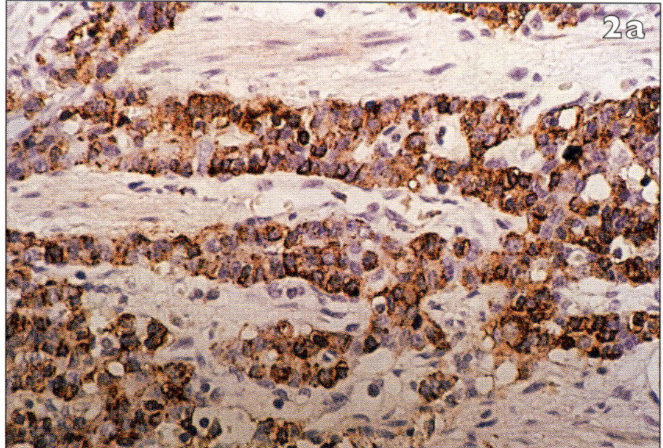

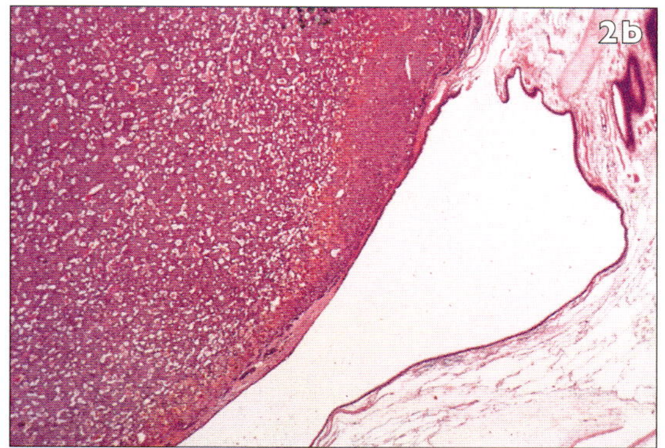

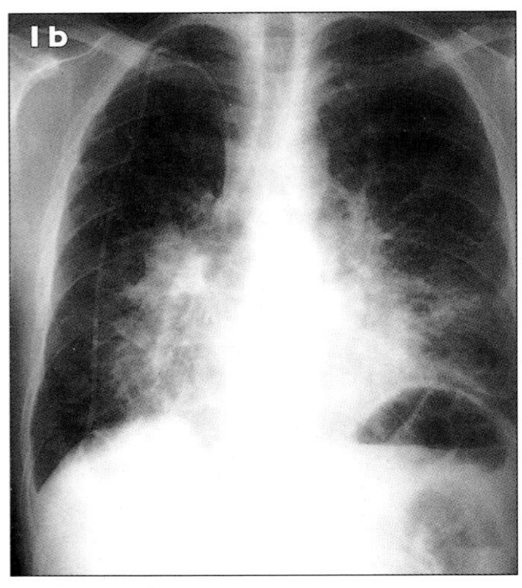

1 i. 1a shows a typical lesion of Kaposi's sarcoma (KS). KS is usually purple but can be red and is either papular or nodular, or less commonly macular or forms plaques. Lymphoedema of the surrounding tissue is often marked. There are often several lesions which can appear at different parts of the body.
ii. KS can remain localized for months or even years in patients with high CD4 counts. Lung involvement is most commonly seen in patients with lower CD4+ lymphocyte counts ($<0.2\times10^9$/l) when the cutaneous lesions often become more widespread and the disease may involve lymph nodes and viscera. Endobronchial involvement can lead to bronchial obstruction with distal collapse or infection. Parenchymal lung disease (1b), often associated with surrounding oedema, may cause dyspnoea with reduced gas transfer. Endobronchial lesions may cause an obstructive pattern on spirometry and frequently present with cough. The chest radiograph can reveal interstitial shadows, nodular shadowing that may coalesce, hilar or mediastinal lymphadenopathy and pleural effusions. Endobronchial lesions may be seen at bronchoscopy. More peripheral or interstitial lesions can be identified on high-resolution CT (spiral) scanning. Localized KS is usually treated with radiotherapy. Cytotoxic drugs such as vincristine and bleomycin or liposomal anthrocycline preparations would be used for disseminated KS, including lung disease.

2 i. The histological features of islands and ribbons of cells with uniform nuclei and cytoplasm are consistent with a carcinoid tumour and the stain chromogranin has been used to verify the neuroendocrine nature of this tumour (2a). Other stains which could have been used for this purpose include neurone-specific enolase and synaptophysin.
ii. The stain is specific for cells of neuroendocrine origin; however, other lung tumours of neuroendocrine origin including small cell carcinoma and atypical carcinoids will also be positive for neuroendocrine staining. Therefore the stain is not specific for carcinoid tumours. Indeed, some non-small-cell tumours may have neuroendocrine components. These stains must therefore be employed along with light microscopy as well as electron microscopy in more difficult cases.
iii. Carcinoid tumours often infiltrate the bronchial wall and the part of it visible at bronchoscopy may be the 'tip of the iceberg'. 2b shows the tumour bulging into the bronchial lumen and deforming it. They also tend to be highly vascular and, if suspected by its macroscopic appearance, are preferably biopsied with rigid bronchoscopy.

3 This low-power photomicrograph (3) of a Wright–Geimsa-stained cytospin has been prepared from bronchoalveolar lavage (BAL) fluid from a normal volunteer.
i. Describe a typical protocol for performing BAL.
ii. What is the expected cell recovery from normal subjects?

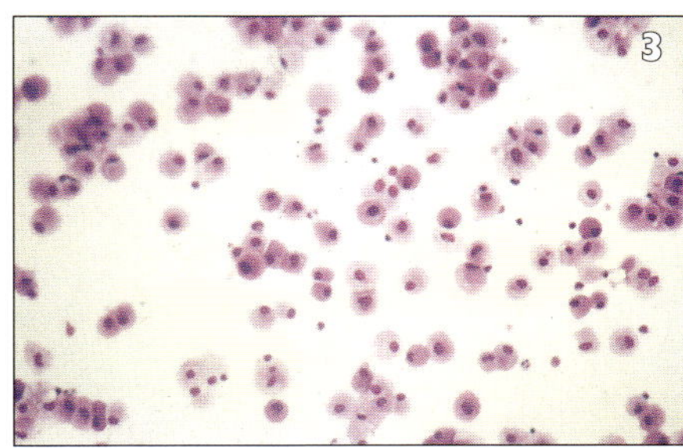

4 i. What is the diagnosis of this transbronchial biopsy (4) and what is the differential diagnosis?
ii. Why is this condition easy to diagnose by transbronchial biopsy?
iii. Which other conditions may be diagnosed confidently by transbronchial biopsy?

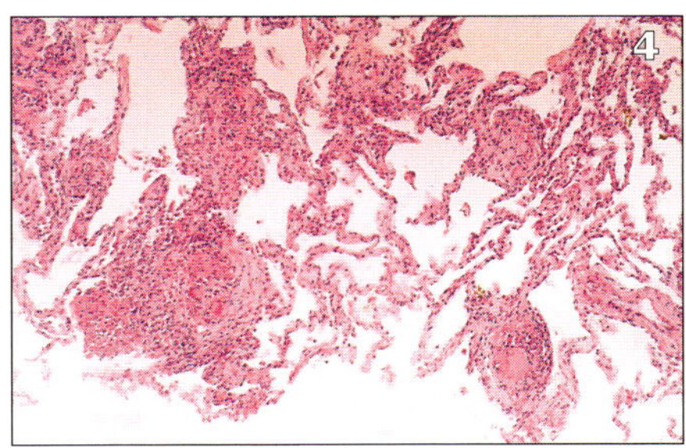

5 The chest radiographs in **5a**, **5b** are of the same 38-year-old man, both taken in full inspiration 2 weeks apart. He presented with ocular symptoms, then bulbar weakness and finally dyspnoea. The vital capacity was 1.2 l. Over the 4 days before the second film was taken he received treatment that required brief daily admissions to the intensive care unit.
i. What is the likely cause of the radiographic abnormalities?
ii. What degree of muscular weakness results in respiratory failure?

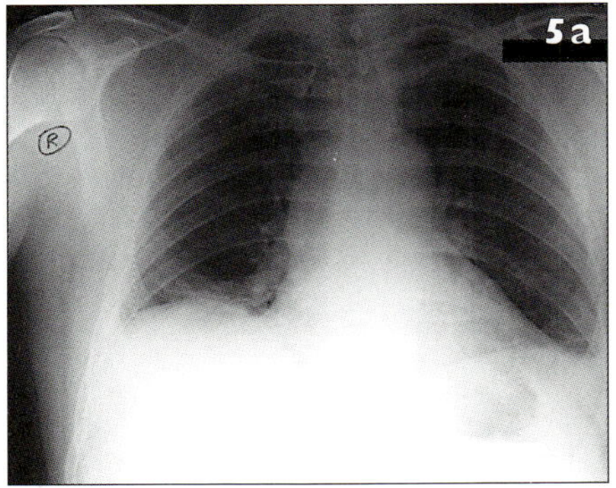

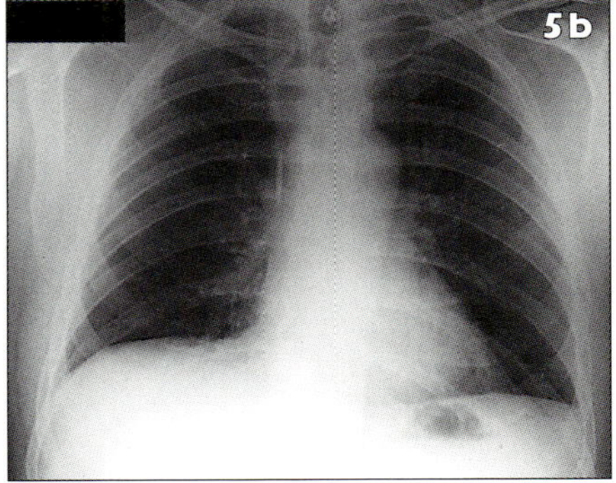

3 i. BAL is performed by wedging the tip of a flexible fibre-optic bronchoscope into a segmental or subsegmental airway until the lumen is occluded. Sequential 30–50 ml aliquots of physiological saline are then instilled through the working channel of the bronchoscope and withdrawn. The total volume of saline used is typically 150–200 ml and approximately 50% is recovered. The remainder is rapidly absorbed or expectorated. It is estimated that BAL fluid represents an approximately 100-fold dilution of alveolar epithelial lining fluid.

ii. Approximately 10×10^6 cells are normally recovered, of which >85% are alveolar macrophages, 7% are lymphocytes (predominantly T-cells), 3% are airway epithelial cells, and <5% each are neutrophils, eosinophils, basophils and mast cells. Greater numbers of cells are commonly found in cigarette smokers and urban dwellers.

4 i. The compact granulomas with a paucity of interstitial inflammation are typical of sarcoidosis.

ii. The granulomas are situated adjacent to bronchi, making them amenable to diagnosis by bronchial or transbronchial biopsy. Only four separate biopsies are usually needed to obtain typical granulomas. A transbronchial lung biopsy may be positive, even when the chest radiograph shows only hilar lymphadenopathy without parenchymal shadowing. The main differential is extrinsic allergic alveolitis, though here the granulomas are not so tightly formed and are overshadowed by an interstitial inflammatory cell infiltrate.

iii. Other conditions which can be readily diagnosed with transbronchial lung biopsy include lymphangitis carcinomatosa and alveolar proteinosis. Conditions such as idiopathic pulmonary fibrosis may be suggested by transbronchial biopsy, but definitive diagnosis usually requires large samples such as from an open lung biopsy.

5 i. The first chest radiograph (**5a**) shows small lung fields with bilateral atelectasis most marked on the right. The second (**5b**) is normal except for the presence of a multiple lumen catheter in the superior vena cava.

ii. The small lung volumes could be due to poor patient effort, but this is, in general, unlikely. A restrictive process should therefore be considered and would include intrapulmonary disease, pleural disease or structural chest wall deformity but there is no radiographic evidence to support these diagnoses. The other possibility is a failure of the muscle pump. As the condition was successfully treated over 2 weeks and the presence of the intravenous catheter noted on the second radiograph suggests the possibility of plasma exchange, it suggests either Guillain–Barré syndrome or myasthenia gravis. The diagnosis was myasthenia gravis.

Acute respiratory failure due to alveolar hypoventilation develops when the vital capacity (VC) falls below 800 ml in an 80-kg individual, but inability to cough and clear secretions would occur earlier. This is particularly relevant when bulbar symptoms are present with the risk of aspiration and pneumonia. The patient had a thymoma and plasma exchange was therefore indicated before surgery.

6 The owner of this bird (6) presented with a 1-week history of cough, fever and myalgia. Her chest radiograph showed patchy shadowing in the right lower zone.
i. What unusual pathogen may be the cause of her illness?
ii. How would you confirm the diagnosis?
iii. What is the treatment of choice?

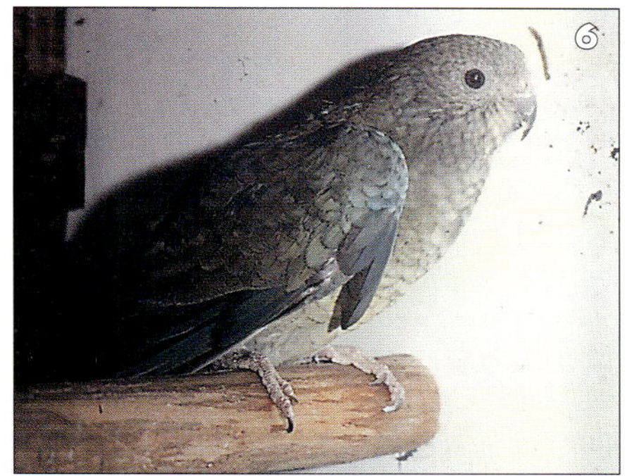

7 As well as dyspnoea, this man also complains of multiple floating spots across his field of vision for several weeks and on examination has retinal haemorrhages and exudates (7a).
i. How commonly would such eye and pulmonary problems be connected?
ii. What is the appropriate management of this situation?

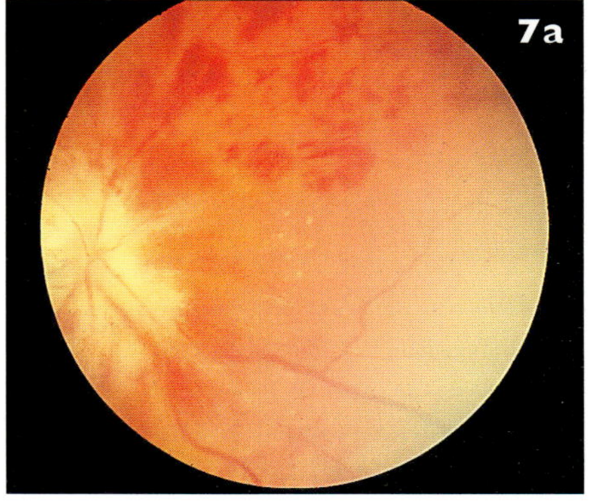

8 This asthmatic man (8) presented acutely with increasing dyspnoea and retrosternal discomfort.
i. What has happened?
ii. How should he be treated?
iii. What other causes of this condition are there?

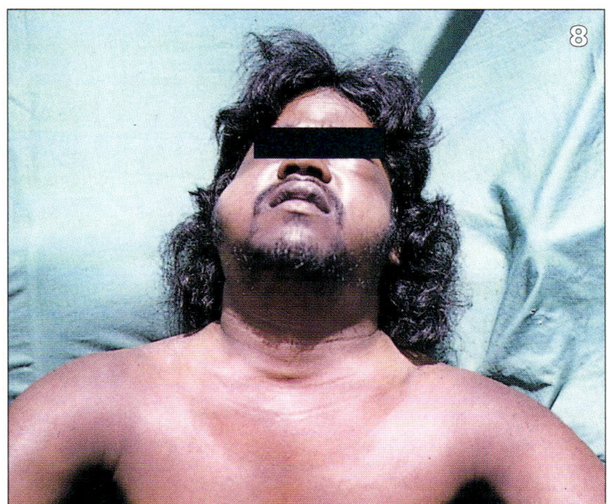

6 i. Infection by *Chlamydia psittaci* (psittacosis) is a possibility, although statistically pneumococcal infection is still most likely. If the bird had been recently acquired or recently bred, or was itself ill, the chances of psittacosis would be increased.
ii. The diagnosis is usually made by serology looking for a four-fold rise in complement-fixing antibodies to the type II antigen of *C. psittaci*. Direct fluorescent staining of respiratory tract secretions can be used to look for chlamydial antigen.
iii. The treatment of choice is tetracycline. A macrolide would be second choice.

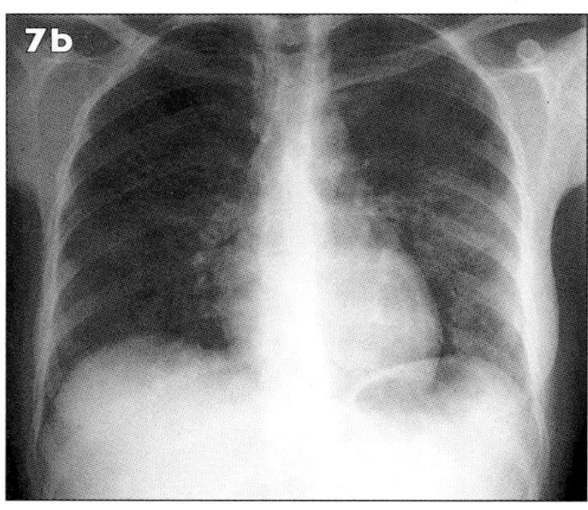

7 i. The retinal problem is due to cytomegalovirus (CMV; 7a). The differential diagnosis of interstitial pneumonitis is as in the answer to **195**, with *Pneumocystis carinii* pneumonitis (PCP) still being the most likely cause (**7b**). Other than the eye, this organism also causes disease of the gut, nervous system and biliary tree. Rarely, CMV may be implicated in HIV-related pneumonitis when other pathogens, such as PCP, have been excluded as a cause.
ii. Initial management would be as in **195**; that is, therapy for presumed PCP until the result of bronchoscopy is obtained. In the rare case of CMV pneumonitis, the patient would be treated with intravenous ganciclovir at high dose for 2–3 weeks. If the CMV pneumonitis occurs without concomitant eye involvement no further therapy is necessary.

8 i. The upper chest and face is grossly swollen. The skin is indented easily and contains palpable crepitus. He has 'surgical' or subcutaneous emphysema. He has either a pneumothorax with mediastinal emphysema which has tracked up and out of the mediastinum, or he has ruptured an airway causing mediastinal emphysema which again has tracked upwards. Usually the condition is self-limiting but can be most uncomfortable and painful especially around the eyes.
ii. A careful check for a pneumothorax should be made with, if necessary, inspiratory and expiratory chest films. Interpretation can be difficult due to extensive extrathoracic gas being present. A CT of the thorax may be necessary. The asthma should be treated as usual. If a pneumothorax is present a large intercostal drain should be inserted. Oxygen should be given by mask to minimize the amount of nitrogen entering the tissues, as nitrogen resorbs more slowly than oxygen.
iii. Other causes include:
- A partially dislodged chest drain; a side hole may become extrathoracic allowing air to pass into the extrathoracic tissues.
- A traumatic pneumothorax with a rib fracture. A chest drain should be inserted and a pressure bandage applied.
- Rupture of a main airway following a deceleration injury or a seat belt injury, which can cause a large pneumo-mediastinum and surgical emphysema.

9 i. Describe the different types of exercise apparatus used for progressive exercise testing.
ii. What is a progressive exercise test and why is it done?

10 i. A 30-year-old man was admitted with fever, cough with haemoptysis and dyspnoea. A few red blood cells but no microorganisms were noted on sputum Gram-stain.
i. What does the lung function test (Table) show?
ii. What does this chest radiograph (**10**) show?
iii. What is the cause?
iv. Name three important conditions associated with this and the laboratory investigations that would differentiate them.

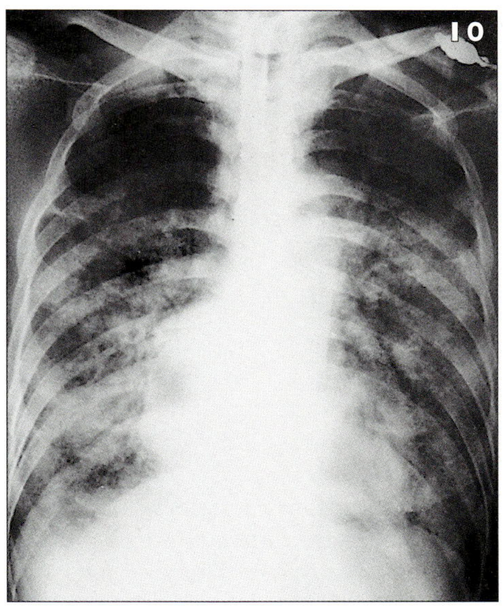

Test	Predicted	Range	Result	% Predicted
PEFR (l/min)	450	383–518	470	104
FEV_1 (l)	2.75	2.34–3.16	1.47	53
FVC (l)	4.05	3.45–4.66	2.23	55
FEV_1/FVC (%)	69	58–79	65	55
DL_{CO} (Hb corrected)[a]	7.88	6.70–9.06	11.07	96
VA (l)	1.47	1.25–1.69	3.72	140
K_{CO} (Hb corrected)[b]	3.09	2.63–3.55	2.97	202

[a]DL_{CO} = transfer factor; [b]K_{CO} = transfer coefficient in DL_{CO}/VA

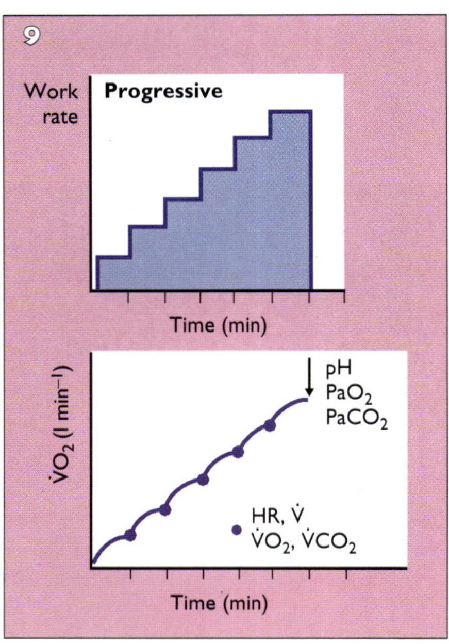

9 i. The different types of apparatus used for progressive exercise tests are a stepping test, or more commonly a treadmill test, or a cycle ergometer test. During these tests, the workload is increased by small increments at regular times. The workload will gradually increase until the patient reaches his/her maximum exercise capacity or maximal oxygen uptake (**9**).

ii. The main purpose of a progressive exercise test is to measure the work capacity achievable by the individual. Several measurements can be made including heart rate, minute ventilation, mixed expired gas concentration by capturing the expired gases with the patient breathing through a two-way valve box via a mouth piece. It is mandatory to measure the ECG during exercise and, from it, the heart rate. Minute ventilation can be measured by collecting expired gas volumes or by sampling the expired gas volumes for the expired CO_2 and oxygen concentration and, from this, the oxygen uptake per unit time (usually minute-by-minute) is measured. The progressive exercise test is commonly used in the investigation of heart disease (e.g. Bruce protocol) where chest pain, ECG abnormalities or breathlessness are looked for. In patients with lung disease, exercise is usually stopped by maximum exercise ventilation being achieved, causing breathlessness. It is also possible to measure arterial blood gases during exercise, either by an indwelling arterial cannula or from arterialized capillary blood collected from an earlobe. Measurements of arterial/arterialized blood gas tensions will allow the alveolar arterial oxygen gradient to be calculated.

10 i. A high K_{CO}, i.e. increased diffusion capacity across the alveolar–capillary membrane. Additional carbon monoxide uptake occurs in the lungs because of the presence of alveolar haemorrhage.

ii. Bilateral alveolar filling pattern.

iii. Pulmonary haemorrhage.

iv. Three important associated conditions and the laboratory investigations that differentiate them are:

- Goodpasture's disease: anti-glomerular basement membrane antibody.
- Wegener's granulomatosis: c-anti-cytoplasmic antibody (c-ANCA).
- Systemic vasculitis: anti-nuclear antibody, anti-double-stranded DNA antibody.

11 This chest radiograph (**11a**) is from a middle-aged man who presented with a cough 3 months after a renal transplant for polycystic kidney disease.
i. What is the differential diagnosis?
ii. How would you investigate this?
iii. What is the treatment of choice?

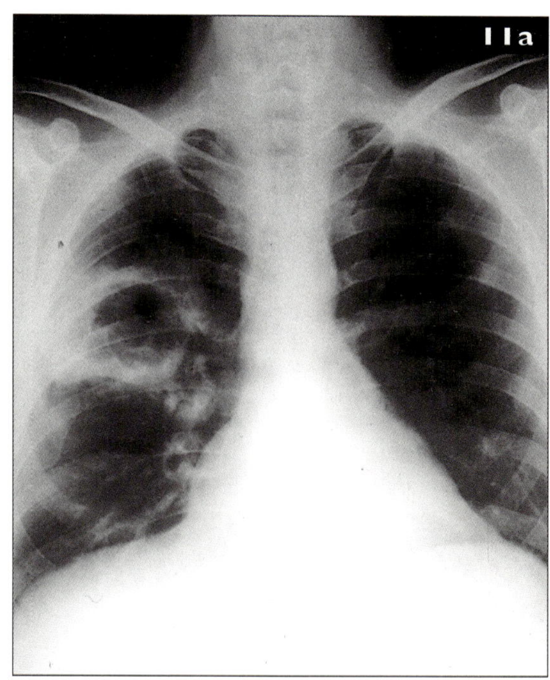

12 This man was referred for consideration of resection of a mass in the left lower lobe. The CT scan (**12**) showed an irregularly shaped lesion with streaky shadowing extending into the depths of the right lower lobe.
i. Of what are these appearances characteristic?
ii. With what are they associated?

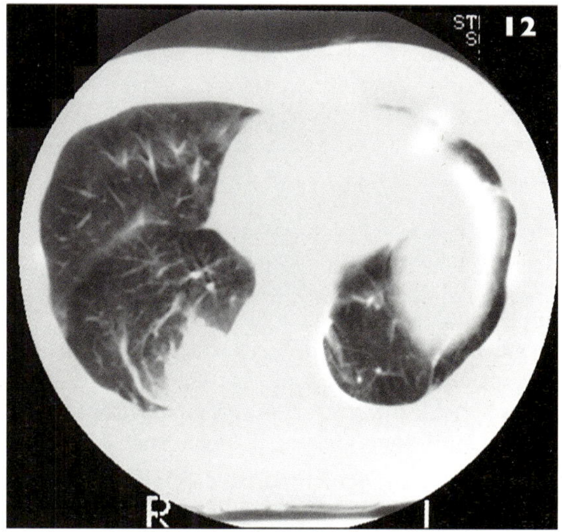

11 i. The chest radiograph shows a large right mid-zone cavity which has a thick, rather irregular wall. Fungal infection, tuberculosis, Gram-negative or anaerobic bacterial infection or a cavitating pulmonary infarct are the most likely causes.
ii. Bronchoscopy with lavage of the affected area, and/or percutaneous needle aspiration of the cavity. CT scanning will delineate the margins of the cavity and its exact position with greater clarity. Recently a halo sign on CT scanning has been suggested to be specific for fungal infection. In this patient both needle aspiration and bronchoscopy revealed *Aspergillus*. **11b** and **11c** are low-power photomicrographs of a histological section of a medium-sized airway obtained at autopsy. Numerous dark-stained branching hyphae can be seen invading the airway wall. Submucosal glands and cartilage are present in the adjacent tissue. Necrotizing aspergillosis can also occur in the larger airways and in the same clinical setting as invasive aspergillosis, although this is less common.

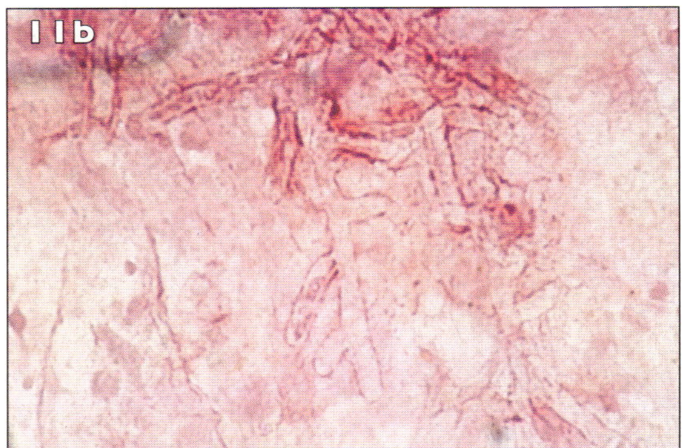

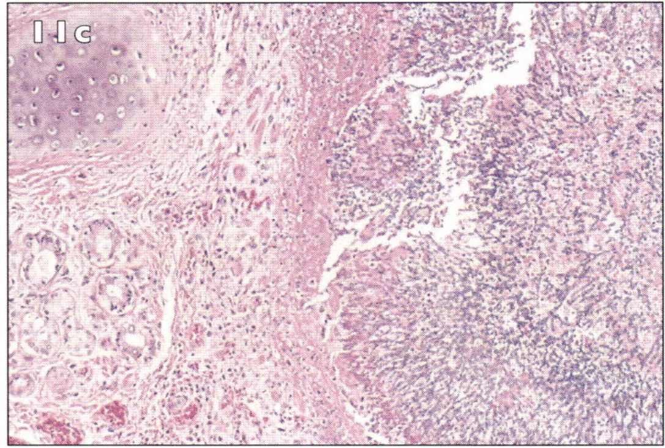

iii. The treatment of choice is intravenous amphotericin, but the prognosis is poor.

12 i. The CT shows a peripheral mass, inseparable from the pleural surface, with tongues of dense tissue that extend medially into the pulmonary parenchyma. This appearance is known as 'folded lung', Blesovsky's syndrome or 'rounded atelectasis'. It is due to part of the dorsal surface of the lung becoming adherent to the parietal pleural surface and causing that segment of the lung to twist and become densely consolidated; this often contains an air bronchogram which can be seen on CT.
ii. This appearance occurs mostly in subjects exposed to asbestos with pleural plaques that become adherent to the visceral pleura, immobilizing the dependent pulmonary segment. The CT appearances are characteristic and require no biopsy or other action.

13 A 24-year-old male motor-cyclist was admitted as an emergency after being involved in a road traffic accident.
i. What abnormality can be seen on the plain chest radiograph (**13a**) and what diagnosis must be suspected?
ii. What is demonstrated on the subsequent vascular imaging films (**13b, 13c**)?
iii. Where is this lesion normally encountered, what is the mechanism of injury and what are the possible consequences?

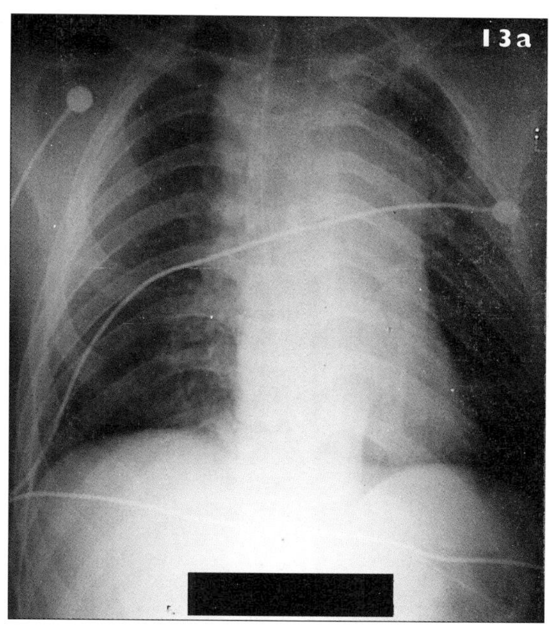

14 A young man presented to the emergency department complaining of left chest pain and breathlessness after a kick to the left side of body.
i. What does the chest radiograph (**14**) show?
ii. What is the differential diagnosis and what surgical treatment should be offered?

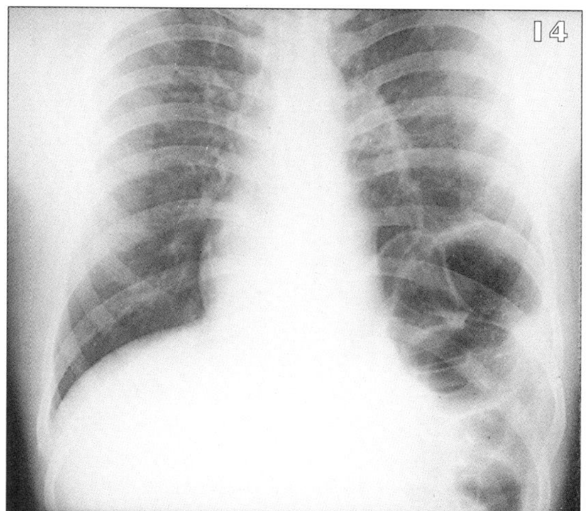

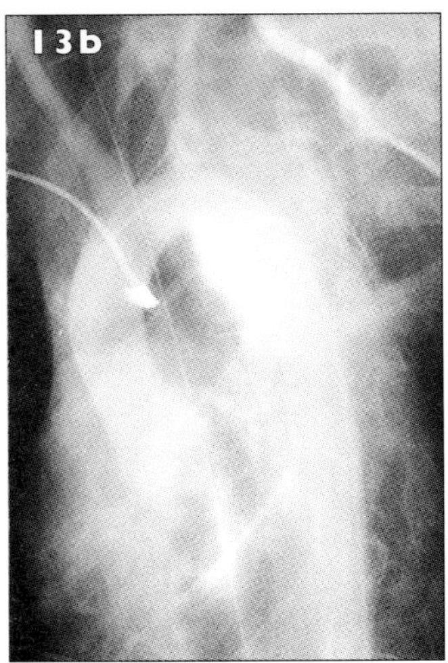

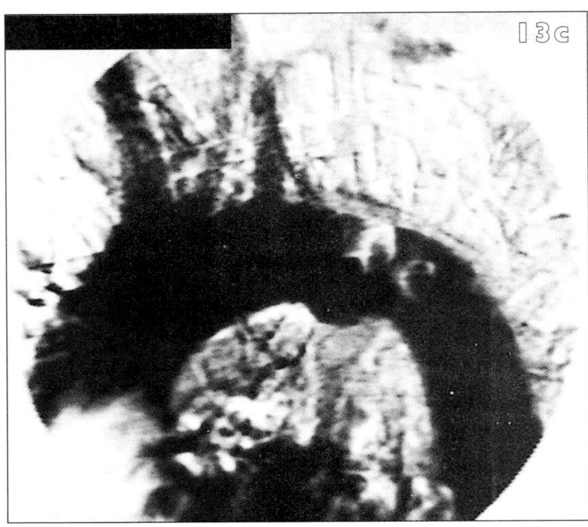

13 i. There is gross widening of the mediastinum on the plain chest radiograph (13a), even allowing for the AP nature of the examination. The severity of the injury and the mediastinal widening make traumatic aortic transection a definite possibility.
ii. The aortogram (13b) shows a bulge in the region of the distal aortic arch/proximal descending aorta. This is clearly shown on digital subtraction angiography (13c) to be due to disruption of the aortic wall.
iii. This lesion is characteristically seen at the aortic isthmus, i.e. the junction between the aortic arch and the descending aorta. This injury is believed to occur because the arch can move forward with deceleration whereas the descending aorta is relatively fixed. Immediate exsanguination will occur in many cases. Those that reach hospital can undergo repair of the ruptured segment, usually with the insertion of a short length of prosthetic graft. Either before or during surgery, spinal cord ischaemia can occur with consequent lower-limb paralysis.

14 i. The left hemithorax contains gas-filled loops of intestine.
ii. The differential diagnosis includes a raised hemidiaphragm, enventration of the diaphragm, congenital diaphragmatic hernia and, given the history of trauma, traumatic rupture of the diaphragm.

Eventration of the diaphragm results from paralysis, hypoplasia or atrophy of the muscle fibres. It can be difficult to diagnose even on CT scan and often is only confirmed at surgery. The aim of surgery in eventration is to incise the thinned-out diaphragmatic leaf and to repair the diaphragm by imbricating one layer over the other. In diaphragmatic hernia or traumatic rupture the diaphragm is repaired either by direct suture or by the placement of a 'patch' (Marlex Mesh) across the defect.

15 This radiograph (15) of a 25-year-old man was taken on admission to hospital via the accident and emergency department. How is ARDS managed?

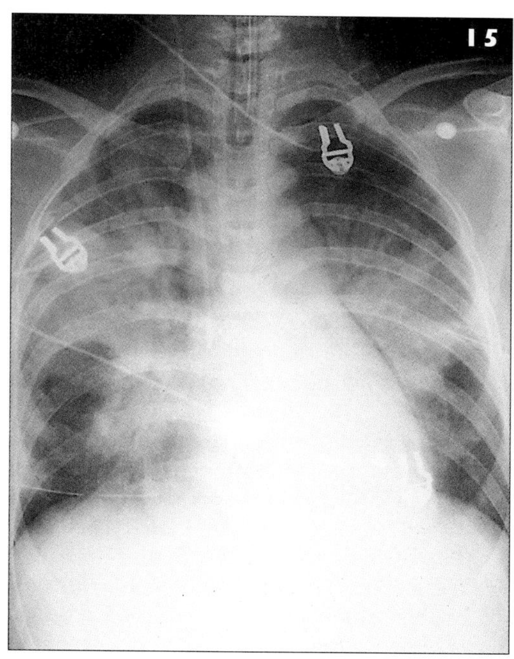

16 Fibreoptic bronchoscopy in this patient revealed a squamous cell carcinoma in the right lower lobe (16). Apart from an increase in dyspnoea, the patient is well. The FEV_1 is 1.8 l. How would you stage for possible thoracotomy?

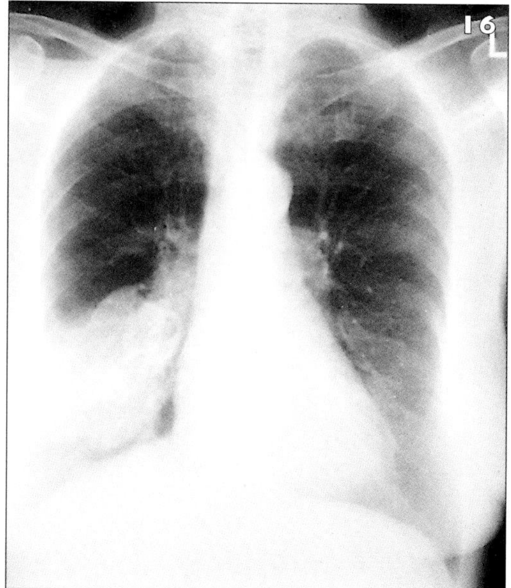

15 The management of ARDS includes:
- Maintenance of adequate arterial oxygen saturations (SaO_2) so that oxygen delivery is not compromised – in this case SaO_2 of 90–92% would be adequate and would allow the inspired oxygen concentrations to be kept below 80% thereby reducing the risks of oxygen toxicity.
- Ventilatory management of ARDS is currently under study – several modes of management have been suggested. In general, none of the newly developed modes have been shown to affect outcome, although recently there has been a trend towards lowering tidal volume (<10 ml/kg) in an attempt to reduce the incidence of barotrauma. Similarly, the levels of PEEP most commonly deployed now seem to be lower than those used 5–10 years ago. Levels that exceed 15 cmH_2O are now rather uncommon. Most recently, 'permissive hypercapnoea' was suggested as a possible alternative approach – controlled trials are currently underway in France and the US.
- It is frequently appropriate to insert a pulmonary artery catheter, both to document the left atrial pressure/wedge pressure and measure cardiac output and oxygen delivery but the complications associated with pulmonary artery catheterization, particularly line-related sepsis, rarely make it appropriate to keep the catheter *in situ* for longer than 48 hours.
- The patient should be well sedated. If the patient is hyperpyrexial, cooling could be considered to minimize oxygen consumption and CO_2 production. On occasions, paralysis may be necessary, but paralytic agents may adversely affect diaphragmatic function.

16 The chest radiograph (**16**) shows consolidation or an intrapulmonary mass with an additional mass at the lower pole of the right hilum. The mediastinum looks normal. Initial tests include a full blood count and biochemical screen. Abnormal liver function tests would require a liver ultrasound or CT to exclude metastases. An elevated serum calcium requires a bone scan, although the primary tumour (if squamous) may cause ectopic secretion of peptide hormones.

If tests are normal, then the only test required is a CT of the thorax and upper abdomen. If this shows no signs of inoperability, the chances of a CT brain or a bone scan identifying an isolated occult metastasis is 1–4%. If the CT thorax shows enlarged mediastinal lymph nodes (>1 cm in their shortest transverse diameter), the final staging investigation should be a mediastinoscopy of the enlarged mediastinal nodes.

17 Parts **a–c** of Figure **17** are segments of a polysomnogram [LEG(R)(L), leg movement; THOR/ABDO RES, thoracic and abdominal movement]. Which of these shows:
i. Obstructive apnoea;
ii. Central apnoea;
iii. Mixed apnoea?

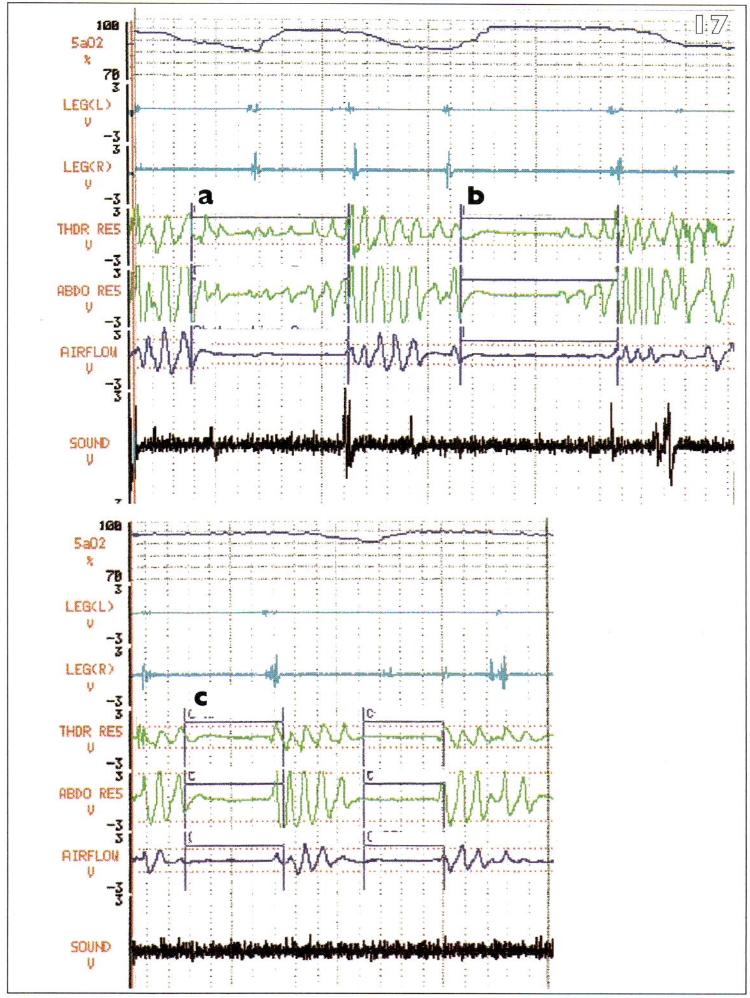

18 i. Describe four distinct clinical presentations of silicosis.
ii. What infection is of particular concern in patients with this disease?

17 i. Obstructive apnoeas (**17a**) are characterized by cessation of airflow with continued evidence of respiratory effort on the chest and abdominal traces, often in a paradoxical fashion. Arterial oxygen saturation decreases during the episodes, periodically reaching a nadir at the end or just after reinitiation of airflow.
ii. Mixed apnoeas (**17b**), a variant of obstructive sleep apnoea, consist of a central event followed by an obstructive portion (respiratory effort begins before airflow does).
iii. Central apnoeas (**17c**) result in a cessation in airflow with no evidence of respiratory effort on the chest and abdominal traces. This event was terminated by an EEG arousal.

18 i. Silicosis is diagnosed by radiographic and clinical criteria in the setting of an appropriate exposure history. The radiographic appearance is classified according to standardized International Labour Office (ILO) criteria. Four distinct forms exist: chronic simple silicosis, progressive massive fibrosis (PMF), accelerated silicosis, and acute silicosis. Chronic simple silicosis is the most common. It is usually recognized as a radiographic abnormality in asymptomatic patients. Small (<1.5 mm) rounded opacities with an upper lobe preponderance slowly develop after 5 to 10 years of exposure. Pulmonary function abnormalities are rare. More severe disease is manifested by more extensive and larger opacities and may be associated with airflow limitation and reduced lung volumes. PMF presents with progressive coalescence of discrete opacities into large, irregular masses, generally in the perihilar regions of the upper lobes. Severe restriction, hypoxaemia, and disabling dyspnoea are often present. The course is often insidious and can progress without ongoing exposure to silica. Accelerated silicosis is uncommon but may develop within 2 to 5 years of intense exposure. In contrast to the upper lobe involvement characteristic of simple silicosis, diffuse, irregular reticulonodular infiltrates are the usual radiographic finding in this form of the disease. The prognosis is poor as progressive disease culminates in death within several years. Acute silicosis occasionally develops following exposure to very high concentrations of silica such as may occur with sandblasting.
ii. Tuberculosis complicating silicosis was first recognized in the 19th century. Silicosis is associated with an increased incidence of infection by *M. tuberculosis* and by atypical mycobacterium. Although symptoms respond readily to therapy, sputum cultures may remain positive. Chronic suppressive therapy with isoniazid following standard multidrug (e.g. isoniazid, rifampicin, pyrizinamide with or without ethambutol) therapy is required in some cases. A tuberculin skin test is mandatory in all patients with silicosis.

19 i. Would you expect any abnormality of the vital capacity of this 18-year-old male patient whose lateral and PA chest radiographs are shown (19a, 19b)?
ii. What associated clinical abnormalities might this patient have?

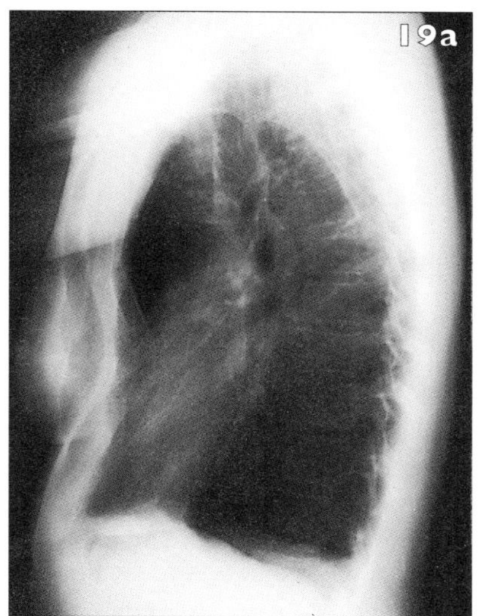
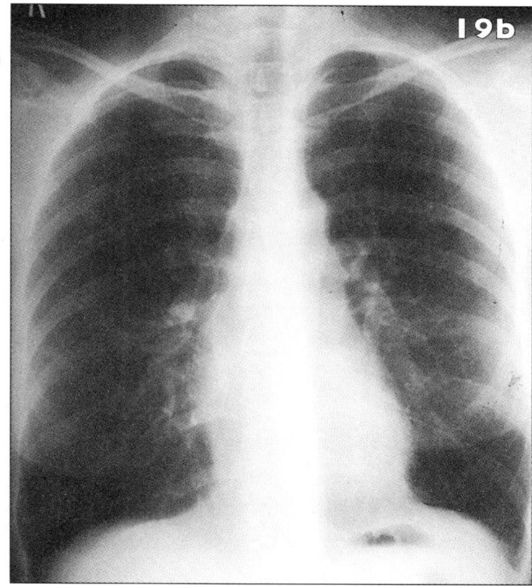

20 A 17-year-old patient complains of paroxysms of sneezing, nasal pruritus, nasal congestion, clear rhinorrhoea and palatal itching. The mucosal surfaces of her eyes and ears were indurated and an examination of her nose revealed a wet reddened mucosa.
i. What is the diagnosis?
ii. What is the treatment?
iii. What are some preventive strategies?

21 i. What is shown in 21?
ii. How does it work?
iii. What is it used for and how useful is it?
iv. What are its side effects?

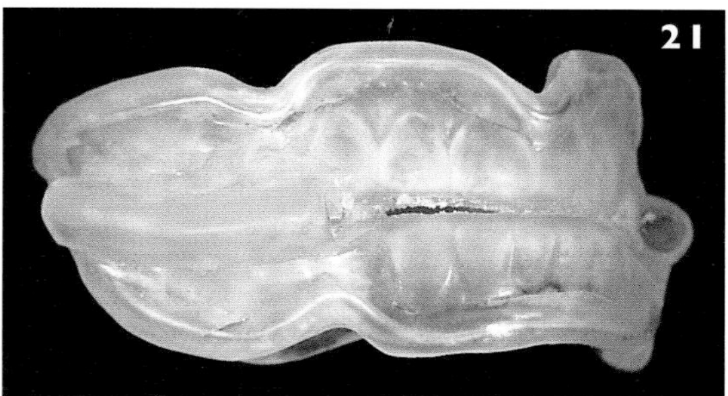

19 i. The lateral chest radiograph (**19a**) shows pectus excavatum, inward displacement of the sternum which has probably been present from birth. Despite what is occasionally a striking physical abnormality it does not cause reduction of the vital capacity, except in a minority of cases. Also, such patients do not have breathlessness due to the sternal deformity.
ii. Associated features include thoracic kyphosis and scoliosis. Cardiac effects include right axis deviation on ECG (due to leftward displacement of the heart), supraventricular tachycardias, mitral valve prolapse and, rarely, reduction of right ventricular filling due to cardiac compression.

20 i. Allergic rhinitis. It is recognized by the greyish appearance of the nasal mucus membranes.
ii. Treatment varies with the severity of the condition but can include some of the following: (a) allergen avoidance; (b) antihistamines for nasal, ocular, and/or palatal itching, and for sneezing and/or rhinorrhoea; (c) nasal topical corticosteroids; (d) oral decongestants in combination with antihistamines; (e) intranasal cromolyn sodium or ipratropium.
iii. The condition may be prevented by avoiding specific antigens (particularly the house dust mite) and by nasal administration of cromolyn. It is also important to exclude the possibility of rhinitis medicamentosa (i.e. overuse of topical nasal α-adrenergic decongestant sprays for more than a few days leading to rebound nasal congestion on withdrawal). Prolonged topical decongestant use might also lead to nasal mucosa hypertrophy and inflammation. When this problem is diagnosed, topical or oral steroids should be initiated as the decongestant spray is tapered.

21 i. A mandibular advancement splint.
ii. Oral appliances are used by dentists for many purposes, including correction of various occlusal disorders. The techniques often modify the position of the mandible within the restricted mobility defined by the temporomandibular joint and the pterygoid muscles. In snoring and obstructive sleep apnoea, these devices are designed predominantly to advance the mandible and pull the base of the tongue forward, thus preventing it from falling backward to occlude the pharynx during sleep.
iii. A review of 21 publications describing 320 patients treated with oral appliances for snoring and obstructive sleep apnoea showed that, despite considerable variation in the design of these appliances, the clinical effects are remarkably consistent. Snoring is improved in almost all patients and is often eliminated. The studies show that OSA improves in the majority of patients. Approximately half of those patients who improve achieve an AHI of <20, but as many as 40% are left with notably elevated AHIs. Sleep is generally improved, although significant sleep disturbance persists in the patients with residual apnoea.
iv. Limited follow-up data indicate that oral discomfort is a common but tolerable side effect, and that dental and mandibular complications appear to be uncommon.

22 The biopsy shown in **22** is from the lower trachea in a 35-year-old male who complained of increasing breathlessness. Chest radiography showed numerous large opacities bilaterally. What is the likely diagnosis?

23 i. Describe the appearances in this chest radiograph (**23**) from a man with a long history of gastrointestinal symptoms.
ii. What are the most likely causative organisms?
iii. What is the treatment of choice?

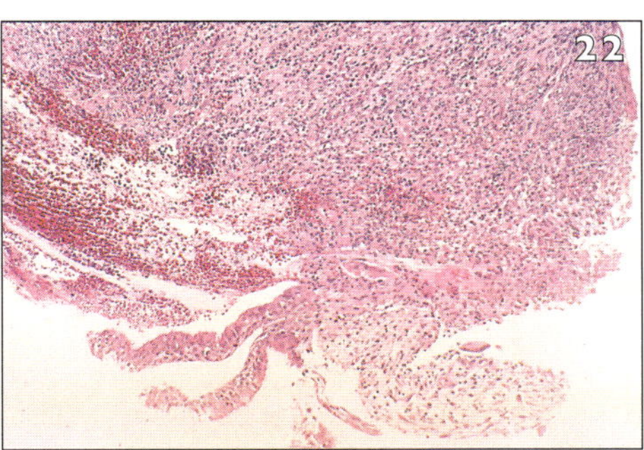

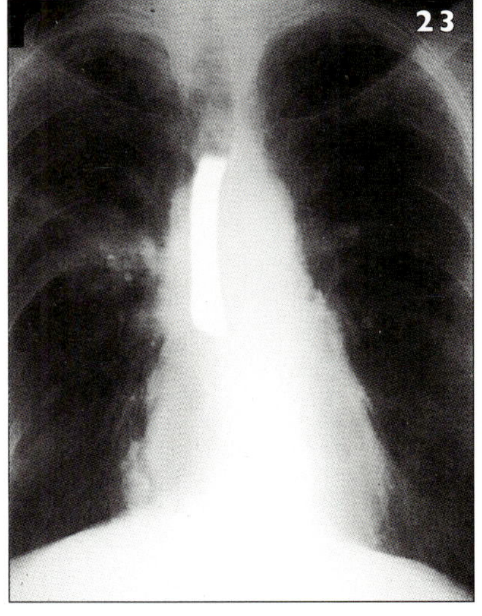

24 This flow–volume loop (**24**) was obtained from a 56-year-old patient with marked respiratory distress and audible wheeze and in whom the initial diagnosis was 'status asthmaticus'. The patient had recently been discharged from hospital after 4 weeks of treatment in intensive care for acute respiratory distress syndrome (ARDS).
i. What does the flow–volume loop demonstrate?
ii. What is the likely diagnosis?
iii. What inhalation treatment might be helpful?

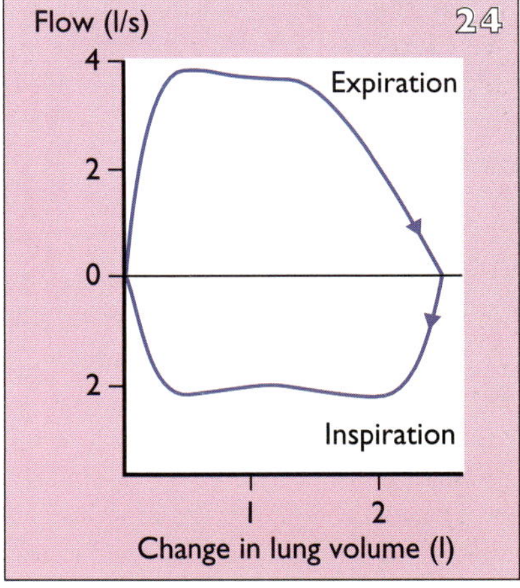

22 There is granulation tissue in the mucosa, and ulceration of the epithelium at the upper left of **22**. These changes are most suggestive of Wegener's granulomatosis. Tracheal and endobronchial involvement are well described in this disease along with lung parenchymal involvement, as manifested by infiltrates or masses on chest radiography. Tracheal involvement may eventually result in stenosis which, if not resolving with anti-inflammatory therapy, may require laser resection. Such therapy may need to be repeated in the event of recurrence. Monitoring endobronchial involvement is best achieved with flow–volume loops and spirometry; the use of anti-neutrophil cytoplasmic antibody titres is less helpful here.

23 i. The chest radiograph shows patchy shadowing in the right mid to upper zone. In the upper mediastinum the oesophagus is outlined by a column of barium, the appearances therefore suggesting oesophageal obstruction and aspiration pneumonia.
ii. The most likely causative organisms would be normal oropharyngeal commensal organisms which are typically anaerobes such as bacteroides or peptostreptococcus. If the patient had spent more than 4 days in hospital before aspiration occurred then Gram-negative enterobacteria would also need to be considered.
iii. The treatment of choice for anaerobic lung infections is either a combination of penicillin plus metronidazole or alternatively, clindamycin. The oesophageal obstruction should also be treated (see **97**).

24 i. The flow–volume loop demonstrates a reduction in the maximum inspiratory and expiratory flows which both plateau over a large proportion of the Force Vital Capacity (FVC) manoeuvre and a low FVC <3 l. The reduction in flow is more marked during inspiration and this is typical of narrowing of the extrathoracic trachea (see **142, 190**).
ii. The initial diagnosis of asthma should be avoided on the basis of the physical signs which, in addition to stridor, are most marked in inspiration but often audible during expiration. A simple test to detect upper airway obstruction (UAWO) is the ratio of FEV_1 to peak flow, i.e. FEVml/PEFR l/min. Normally this is less than 10 but in UAWO the peak flow is affected most, e.g. 2000 ml/150 l/min = 13.
The data would be compatible with a high tracheal or laryngeal area of narrowing/collapse, the most likely cause in this case is tracheal narrowing following a tracheostomy due to a mass of friable granulation tissue at the tracheostomy site. This was the diagnosis and the problem was effectively treated by diathermy.
iii. A mixture of oxygen (21%) and helium (79%) as helium is less dense than nitrogen, allowing greater flow of gas.

25 A 57-year-old non-smoking man, with no respiratory symptoms, began to behave in an uncharacteristically aggressive and uninhibited manner early in the morning. What is the likely cause of the radiograph shadow (**25**) and what is the explanation of his behaviour?

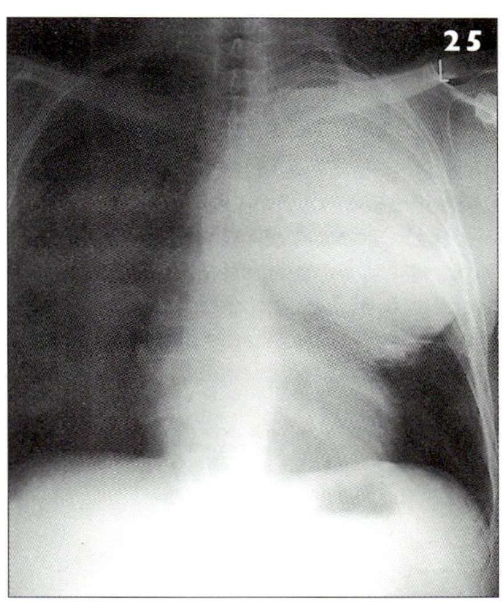

26 A 20-year-old patient complained of severe breathlessness each time after he roller-blades. The result of exercise testing revealed is shown in **26**.
i. What does the exercise test show?
ii. What is the diagnosis?
iii. How would you manage this condition?
iv. What is the pathogenesis of this condition?
v. What drugs are allowed by the Olympic committee before competition?

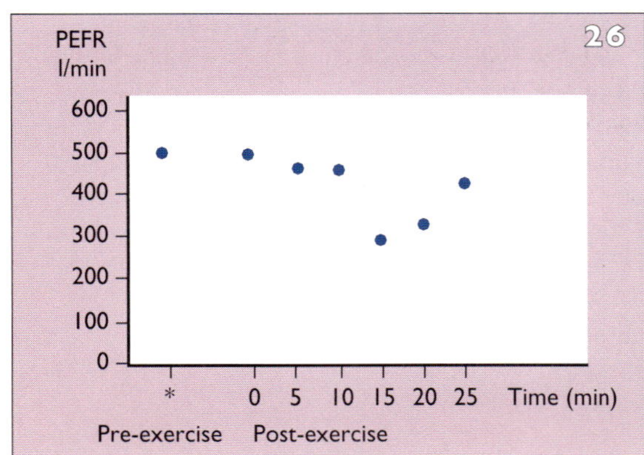

27 This worker (**27**) is properly attired to perform sandblasting safely.
i. Which pneumoconiosis is associated with this occupational exposure?
ii. What other occupations pose similar risks?

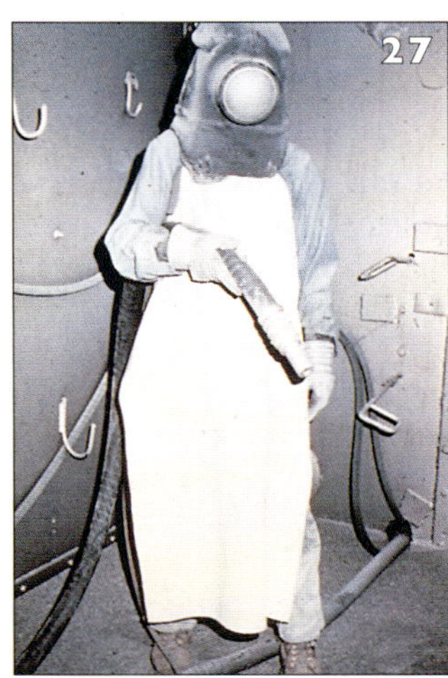

25 Massive pleural fibroma, with spontaneous hypoglycaemia. The huge size of the tumour in an otherwise healthy patient suggests that it is benign in nature. The diagnosis is easily confirmed by percutaneous needle biopsy. Large mesenchymal tumours may produce insulin-like growth factors. It is probable that these peptides both stimulate the growth of the tumour itself, which may attain great size, and lead to spontaneous hypoglycaemia. Insulin-like growth factors are normally produced under the control of growth hormone and their abnormal production leads to its suppression by a negative feedback mechanism. Plasma insulin and C-peptide levels are also low. Despite their large size, these tumours can be removed quite easily surgically as they usually arise from the parietal pleura on a finger-like stalk. Resection leads to complete resolution of the biochemical abnormalities.

26 i. A 40% fall in peak flow reading after exercise compared with pre-exercise value.
ii. Exercise-induced asthma. This diagnosis requires a minimum change of 25% in PEFR from the pre-exercise value to the lowest measurement – usually found 10–20 minutes post-exercise.
iii. Advise the patient to inhale beta-agonist 15 minutes before exercise and to warm-up adequately.
iv. Exercise results in isocapnic hyperventilation and inhalation of cold air which results in water loss from the airway lining, causing airway cooling and hypertonicity. These result in vasoconstriction and mast-cell activation and stimulation of the neural reflexes which cause rebound vasodilatation, oedema and bronchial hyperreactivity. Mucosal thickening and smooth muscle contraction will then occur, leading to bronchoconstriction of the airways. Current research shows that leukotrienes may also play an important role in exercise-induced asthma.
v. Beta-agonists and sodium cromoglycate.

27 i. Silicosis is a chronic, fibronodular interstitial lung disease caused by inhalation of free crystalline silica (SiO_2). Silica occurs both complexed with other elements and in isolation as a 'free' form. The latter, occurring primarily as quartz, tridymite and cristobalite are associated with fibrotic lung disease. Tridymite and cristobalite are more fibrogenic than quartz.
ii. Sandblasting is widely used to clean and etch stone and metal surfaces. Highly pressurized air or water drives a stream of abrasive sand into the workpiece. Very high concentrations of respirable silica are present in the resulting dust cloud. Non-siliceous particulates are increasingly used to minimize this risk, but if the target surface (e.g. stone) contains silica, significant exposure may still occur. Because silica is a major constituent of the earth's crust, mining, tunnelling, quarrying and stone cutting may also entail significant exposure to silica-containing dust. Finely powdered quartz, known as silica flour or tripoli, is another common source of exposure as it is used as a polishing agent, as a dry lubricant in the rubber industry and as a thickening agent in paints and plastics.

28 These arterial blood gas tensions (Table) are from a 25-year-old man with nocturnal confusion 24 hours after the pinning of a fractured femur sustained in a motor vehicle accident. No abnormality was detected on physical examination or chest radiography. What is the likely diagnosis and management?

Test	Result	Reference Range
FIO_2	0.3	–
pH	7.54	7.35–7.45
pCO_2	3.7 kPa (28 mmHg)	4.6–6.0 (35–46mmHg)
pO_2	9.1 kPa (69 mmHg)	12–16 (91–122mmHg)
HCO_3	18 mmol/l	22–30

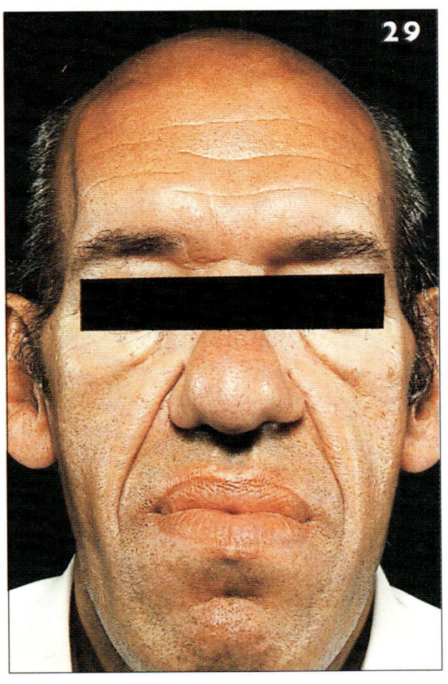

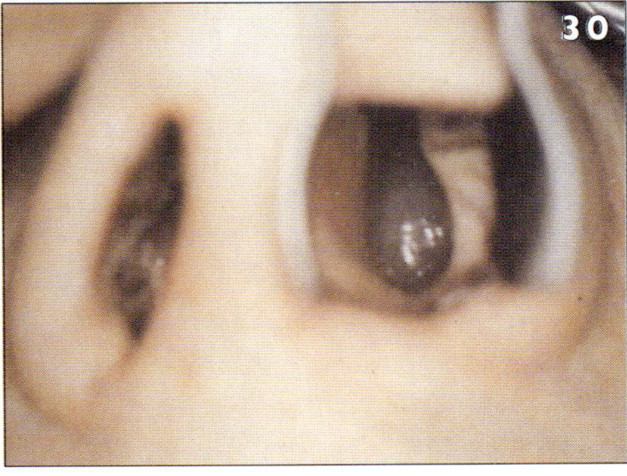

30 i. What condition is seen in **30**?
ii. How is it treated?
iii. What is the common association of this when it occurs in patients with asthma?

29 i. What is the cause of this patient's (**29**) obstructive sleep apnoea?
ii. How would you treat this condition?
iii. If the sleep apnoea is severe, what precaution would you take prior to and after surgery?

28 Fat embolism syndrome. Acute lung injury arises due to deposition of fat globules displaced from the marrow of the fractured bone into the pulmonary arteries, with subsequent release of free fatty acids. The syndrome begins with tachypnoea very soon after the trauma or orthopaedic surgery. Chest radiographs may initially be normal but may progress to show a pattern of acute respiratory distress syndrome, at which time chest examination will reveal widespread fine crackles. Treatment is with oxygen and is supportive as for any other form of acute lung injury. Corticosteroids are of no benefit, except possibly if given early. Other features of the syndrome include central nervous system effects ranging from mild disorientation to seizures and coma, usually 12–36 h after injury. Petechiae may be present, particularly in the conjunctivae and over the upper extremities and axillae. Both of these features are the result of microvascular injury.

29 i. Acromegaly – there is typical frontal bossing with prominent supraorbital ridges, prognathism, coarse skin and thickened lips. Another endocrinological cause for obstructive sleep apnoea is myxoedema.
ii. Transphenoidal removal of the pituitary gland. Octreotide, which is a somatostatin analogue, has also been reported to improve obstructive sleep apnoea in some patients with acromegaly. Despite successful surgery, most acromegalic patients continue to have significant sleep apnoea which requires treatment with nasal CPAP.
iii. The patient should be put on nasal CPAP before and immediately after surgery, even if the surgery is potentially curative. This is because anaesthesia and opiates can cause a further reduction in upper airway tone and a suppression of their arousal response to obstruction. Once the patient has recovered from the surgery, a repeat sleep study should check whether there is still significant obstructive sleep apnoea.

30 i. A nasal polyp, a red mass in the region of the middle turbinate. These occur when oedematous sinus mucosa prolapses into the nasal cavity. They are often associated with perennial rhinitis and low-grade sinusitis.
ii. Nasal polyposis should be treated medically with a short course of oral steroids or local steroid drops followed by topical steroid sprays. If this is not successful, intranasal or endoscopic polypectomy can be considered for polyps that occlude the nasal cavity. Surgery is not curative, however, and the recurrence rate is greater than 40%. For polyposis that occurs in the setting of chronic rhinosinusitis the allergic disease should be treated with antihistamines, topical nasal corticosteroids and immunotherapy.
iii. Some 20–40% of patients with asthma have nasal polyps and many of these patients are allergic to aspirin; 10% of all chronic asthmatics respond to aspirin or other non-steroidal anti-inflammatory drugs with an exacerbation of asthma and acute rhinoconjunctivitis. Some 30% of asthmatics with polypoid rhinosinusitis have aspirin sensitivity.

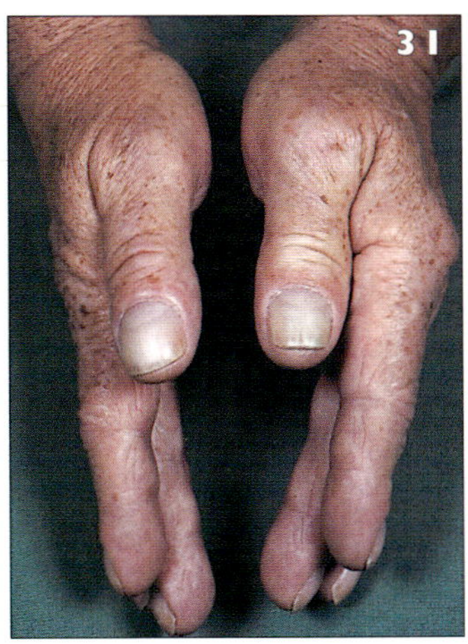

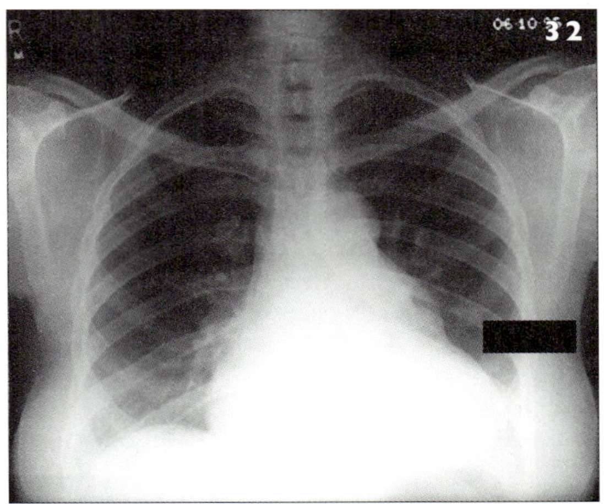

31 Shown (31) is a para-malignant syndrome.
i. What is this condition? How can the arms and legs be affected and how is the latter recognized?
ii. With what else is it associated?

32 What is the major abnormality on this chest radiograph (32)? What further investigations should be carried out to investigate this abnormality?

33 Lung function data are shown in the Table for a patient with rheumatoid arthritis on low-dose methotrexate. The lung function was normal when the drug was commenced 2 months previously and a chest radiograph showed bilateral alveolar shadowing. Could the abnormalities be due to methotrexate?

Test	Predicted	Range	Result	% predicted
FEV_1 (l)	3.32	2.83–3.82	2.24	67
FVC (l)	4.17	3.54–4.79	2.53	61
FEV_1 (%)	81	68–93	88	110
FRC (l)	3.53	3–4.06	1.7	48
TLC (l)	5.8	4.93–6.67	3.34	58
VC (l)	4.17	3.54–4.79	2.23	54
RV (l)	1.6	1.36–1.84	1.11	69
DL_{CO} (mmol/min/kPa)[a]	9.58	8.14–11.02	5.87	61
VA(l)	–	–	3.05	–
K_{CO} (mmol/min/kPa/l)[b]	1.88	1.6–2.16	1.92	100

[a]DL_{CO} = transfer factor; [b]K_{CO} = transfer coefficient in DL_{CO}/VA.

31 i. The hands show clubbing with loss of nail fold angles. This is associated with non-small-cell lung cancers. It can be associated with pain and swelling of the distal forearm and shins which can become red, oedematous and the bones themselves very tender to pressure. Radiography will show new bone formation or periostitis. The condition is known as hypertrophic pulmonary osteoarthropathy (HPOA). Treatment is with non-steroidal anti-inflammatory medication and, if possible, treatment of the primary tumour.

ii. HPOA occurs primarily with lung cancer but has also been reported in association with pulmonary sepsis, thymic carcinoma, chronic myeloid leukaemia, thyroid carcinoma, Hodgkin's disease, adenocarcinoma of the oesophagus, primary lymphocarcinoma of the lung and bronchial carcinoid tumour. Benign associations include cyanotic congenital heart disease, pleural fibroma, Grave's disease, oesophageal achalasia, portal cirrhosis, inflammatory bowel disease, leioma of the oesophagus, cystic fibrosis and idiopathic or familial HPOA.

32 The left heart border is obscured by an opacification which protrudes in the aortopulmonary area. The features are consistent with an anterior mediastinal mass but the differential diagnosis includes a large left atrial appendage.

Further investigation should consist of a CT scan to delineate the extent of any mediastinal mass. If the abnormality arises from the heart or pericardium, lateral chest radiography and then further investigation by echocardiography should be carried out. In this case the abnormality was confirmed, on CT scan, to be a large anterior mediastinal mass which descended to involve the pericardium; it surrounded all the great vessels including the arch of the aorta. Following confirmation of the presence of a large anterior mediastinal mass, subsequent investigation should be by left anterior mediastinotomy, to obtain tissue for histological diagnosis. Mediastinoscopy is not indicated because the arch of the aorta would prevent adequate exposure of the mass for biopsy by this approach. Histological diagnosis revealed an enlarged thymus gland with lymphoid hyperplasia and cyst formation.

33 The lung function data suggest a moderately severe restrictive defect with reduced gas transfer and this, along with the radiographic picture, suggests an acute pneumonitis, which has been associated with the use of methotrexate. The pathogenesis may be either a hypersensitivity or an idiosyncratic drug reaction. In general, elderly patients and those with poor renal function (reducing renal drug clearance) are at risk of methotrexate side effects. Data on lung function disturbances with methotrexate are confounded as patients with rheumatoid arthritis develop interstitial shadowing and opportunistic infections. Indeed, *P. carinii* pneumonia should always be excluded in both suspected acute or chronic toxicity before assuming that the drug is the cause. Lung biopsy findings in methotrexate lung toxicity range from lymphocytic infiltrates to interstitial fibrosis. Milder cases usually respond to stopping therapy; however, corticosteroid therapy would be warranted in the case described here.

34 This is a chest radiograph (34) from a 45-year-old man who presented with a 2-week history of cough, fever and sweats.
i. Describe the appearances.
He was treated with an aminopenicillin for a week but with no influence on his symptoms and he was referred to hospital.
ii. What simple test could confirm the clinical diagnosis?
iii. What is the treatment of choice?

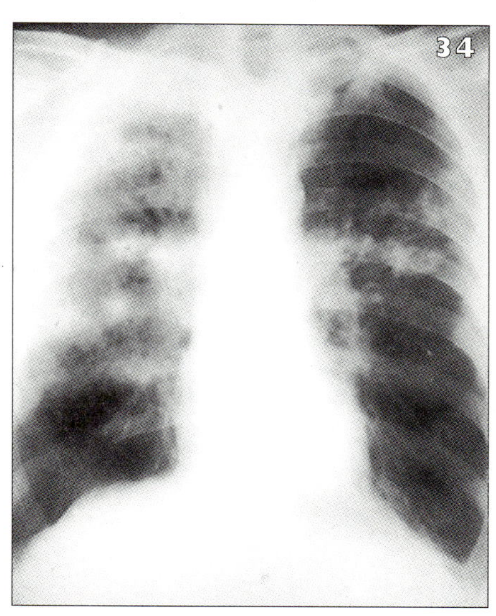

35 What are the indications for use of each of these three oxygen delivery devices (35) in the acute setting?

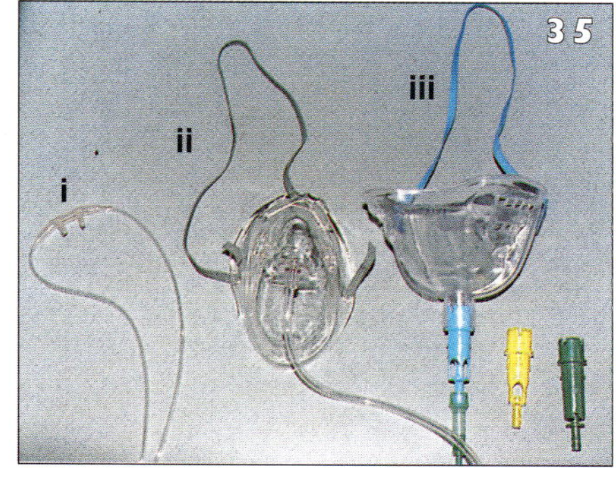

36 This scan (36) was taken 5 years after the patient, a 55-year-old man, presented with a blood-stained pleural effusion. At that time examination of the fluid and bronchoscopy were negative. What is the abnormality shown and what are the possible causes?

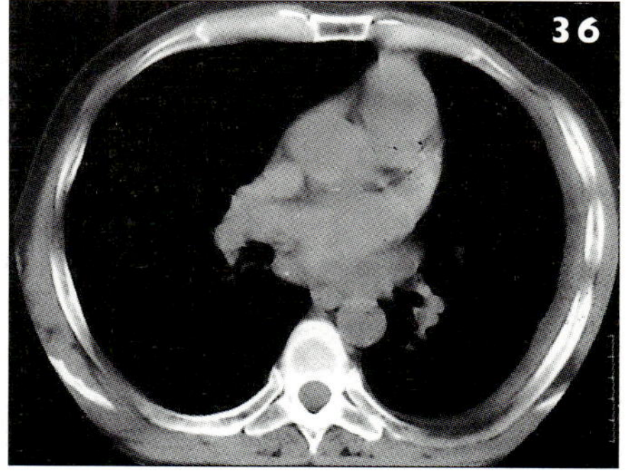

34 i. The chest radiograph (**34**) shows the presence of patchy shadowing in the right upper and mid-zones with smaller area of shadowing in the left mid-zone.
ii. Ziehl–Nielsen stain of the patient's sputum showed the presence of acid-fast bacilli, confirming the clinical suspicion of tuberculosis. Tuberculosis can mimic simple community-acquired pneumonias, although the symptom duration is usually longer and patients usually lack the acute toxic features of a bacterial pneumonia.
iii. The treatment of choice is with combination anti-tuberculous chemotherapy which in a population at low risk of resistant organisms should be with three drugs (rifampicin, isoniazid and pyrazinamide) for 2 months followed by two drugs (rifampicin and isoniazid) for a further 4 months. A fourth drug should be added initially in those at risk of resistant organisms, e.g. those of ethnic minorities or who have had previous treatment for tuberculosis.

35 i. Nasal prongs are useful at flow rates of 2–3 l/min for mild hypoxaemia.(SaO_2 <88–90%). They allow the patient to eat or drink and there is no CO_2 re-breathing. Higher flow rates can be achieved, although this may cause discomfort and dry the nasal mucosa and the inspiration of oxygen delivered is variable and uncontrolled and therefore potentially harmful.
ii. Hudson, or MC face mask. These can deliver oxygen at flow rates up to 15 l/min corresponding to an approximate FiO_2 of 0.7. The amount of delivered oxygen is dependent on the rate and depth of the patient's respiration and is not safe in patients with reduced hypoxic drive who require controlled oxygen therapy.
iii. Venturi mask. This enables controlled oxygen (24, 28, 35%) to be delivered at high flow rates. Entrainment of air occurs through the holes in the coloured fittings at the neck of the mask to give the high total flow rate which may be needed in severely dyspnoeic patients. It is indicated in hypoxaemic patients with reduced hypoxic drive where oxygen delivery must be constant to prevent uncontrolled respiratory depression with subsequent hypercapnia. A range of fittings is available giving a range of inspired oxygen concentrations. Each fitting requires a different oxygen flow rate from the wall oxygen outlet.

36 Benign pleural thickening. In contrast to the scan of malignant pleural mesothelioma, the pleural thickening is smooth and diffuse, with only slight constriction of the hemithorax. A blood-stained pleural effusion is always suggestive of malignancy, but the long history makes this unlikely and this case was, in fact, due to benign asbestos-related pleurisy. CT-guided needle biopsy showed only hyalinized fibrous tissue, with no evidence of tumour and the patient remains in good health 5 years later with only mild dyspnoea of effort.

Diffuse asbestos-related pleural fibrosis usually follows organization of episodes of pleurisy with effusion and is often bilateral. It tends to progress slowly, leading to a constrictive defect of ventilation with reduction in static and dynamic lung volumes and increasing dyspnoea, but the gas transfer factor remains normal or may be elevated. There is a significant incidence of malignant mesothelioma developing at a later stage and the patient should be followed-up regularly.

37 i. What does the open lung biopsy in **37** show?
ii. What is its pathogenesis?
iii. What conditions predispose to this appearance?

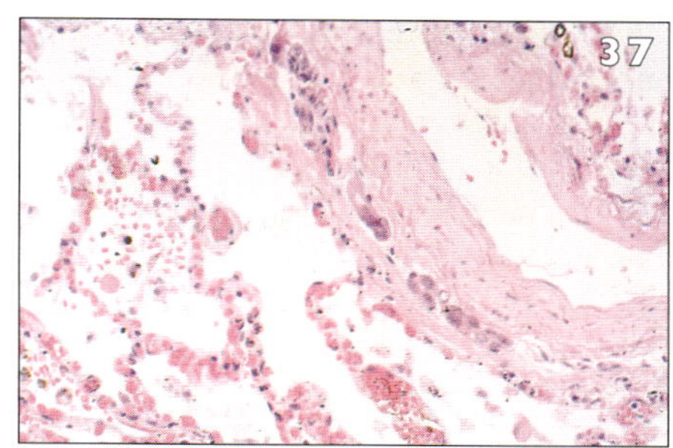

38 Enumerate types of mediastinal involvement by lung cancer and how they may present. What is the cause of this radiological appearance (**38**)?

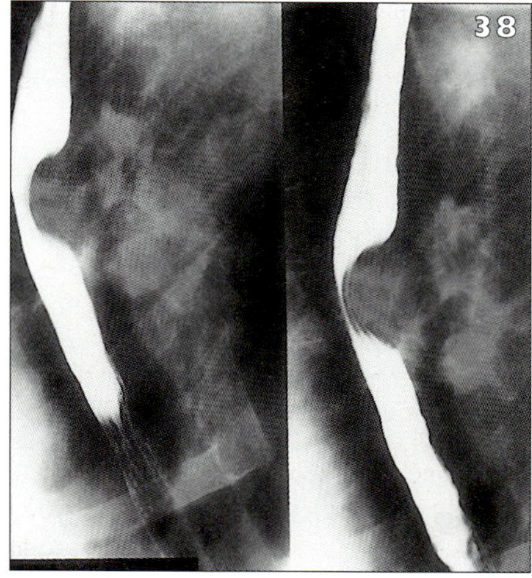

39 A patient with bronchial asthma has persistent nocturnal attacks of cough and wheezy breathlessness which are not controlled despite inhaled steroid therapy and long-acting beta-2 agonists. The cause of the nocturnal attacks was found when 24-hour oesophageal pH monitoring (**39**) was done.
i. What is the cause of the persistent nocturnal attacks?
ii. How can this patient's asthma be controlled?

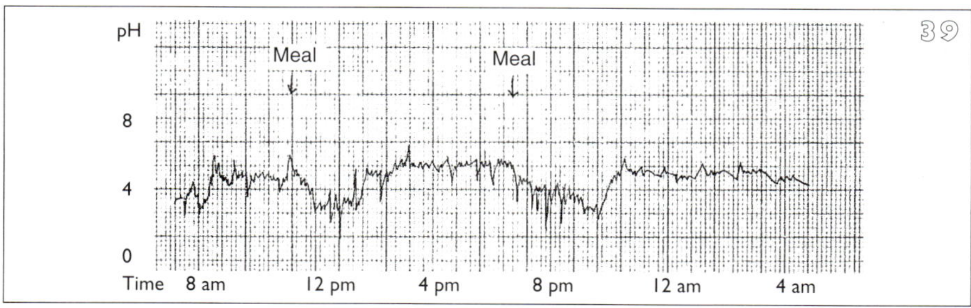

37 i. The lymphatic channels next to the large vessel are infiltrated by tumour cells. There is some vascular congestion. Both are typical of lymphangitis carcinomatosa.
ii. Tumour enters the lungs via the pulmonary arteries and embeds in the vessel wall from where it penetrates into the adjacent lymphatics with subsequent permeation throughout the lung. Some patients may only have spread within the vascular tree. Marked reduction in carbon monoxide gas transfer may be demonstrated in these cases of vascular permeation.
iii. The most common tumour that gives rise to this condition is adenocarcinoma; primary sites include breast, stomach, prostate, ovary, endometrium, pancreas and colon. When these tumours are known to be present the diagnosis is relatively simple. However, lymphangitis carcinomatosa may be the presenting symptom of these tumours so the cause of breathlessness may be confused with pulmonary oedema or benign causes of interstitial lung disease until transbronchial or open lung biopsy is performed.

38 Mediastinal involvement includes:
- Left recurrent laryngeal nerve palsy presents as hoarseness, and poor cough. It is due to metastases in the subaortic fossa.
- SVCO is caused by tumour compression by the right paratracheal lymph nodes.
- Dysphagia can be due to mediastinal lymphadenopathy of the subcarinal nodes. Barium swallow identifies the location of the obstruction (38).
- Arrhythmias, usually atrial fibrillation, can be caused by direct pericardial invasion by tumour, particularly from the left lower lobe.
- Pericardial effusion – as above, is due to direct invasion by tumour. Tamponade can ensue with dyspnoea and appropriate physical signs.
- High hemidiaphragm due to phrenic nerve entrapment in the mediastinum.

Horner's syndrome results, usually, from a primary apical tumour extending on to the posterior mediastinal surface entrapping the sympathetic chain. It is characterized by a small pupil with enophthalmos on the affected side. There is partial ptosis due to paralysis of the sympathetically innervated portion of orbicularis occulis muscle (Muller's muscle). Also, there is unilateral absence of sweating on the face and forehead.

39 i. Gastro-oesophageal reflux. This figure shows numerous episodes of increased oesophageal acidity, especially after meals. Continuous oesophageal pH monitoring can yield a temporal profile of acid reflux and acid clearance. Variables for measurement include the number of reflux episodes, acid clearance times and oesophageal exposure to acid. Possible pathophysiological factors include reflex vagal bronchoconstriction due to nerve fibre stimulation in the lower oesophagus and microaspiration.
ii. In addition to an inhaled steroid and a beta-agonist, oesophageal reflux should be minimized by instructing the patient to sleep with the head elevated, take smaller but more frequent meals, and to take regular H_2 receptor antagonists and motility drugs. The patient should also avoid factors which can reduce the gastro-oesophageal sphincter tone such as caffeine, chocolate, cigarette smoking and medication such as theophylline.

40 i. What abnormality is shown on this radiograph (**40**)?
ii. What is the differential diagnosis?
iii. What additional radiological study can be done to assess the abnormality?

41 i. The material in **41** was obtained from whole lung lavage of a patient with what disorder?
ii. What is the appropriate treatment for this condition?
iii. Do corticosteroids have a therapeutic role?

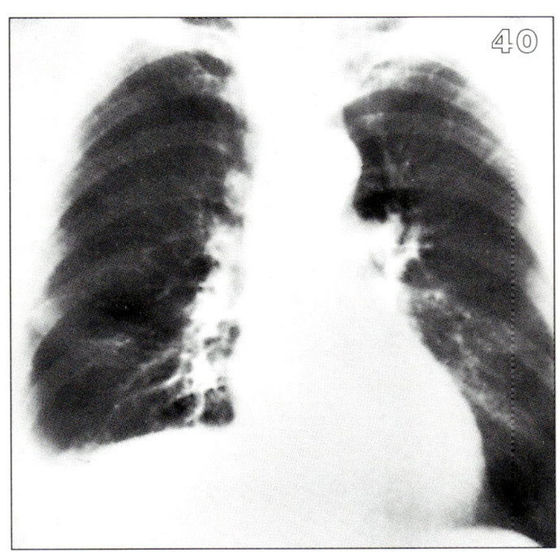

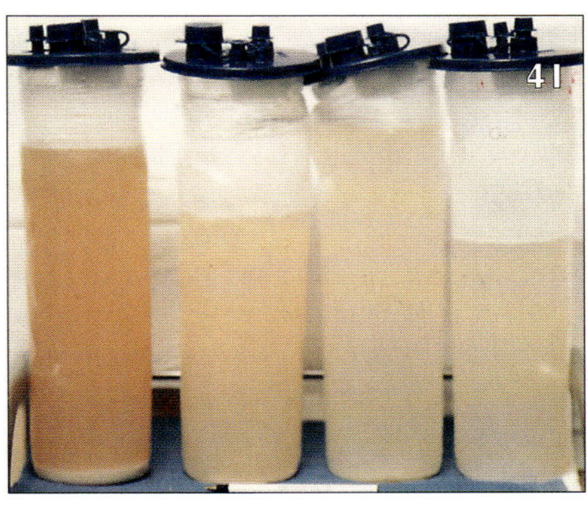

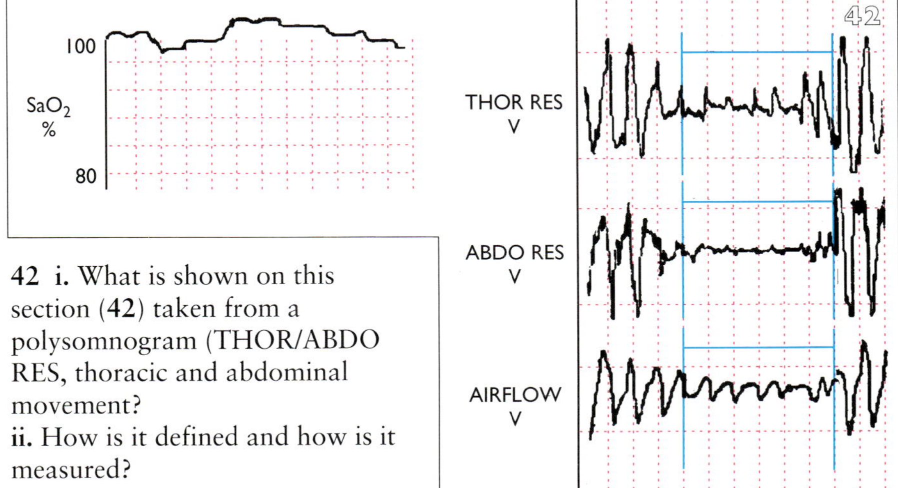

42 i. What is shown on this section (**42**) taken from a polysomnogram (THOR/ABDO RES, thoracic and abdominal movement?
ii. How is it defined and how is it measured?

40 i. The radiograph (40) demonstrates unilateral diaphragmatic elevation.
ii. This problem is most commonly caused by phrenic nerve paralysis. The nerve originates from the third, fourth, and fifth cervical roots. The most common causes of phrenic nerve paralysis include: (a) invasion by bronchogenic carcinoma; (b) disruption from thoracic trauma; (c) cold thermal injury associated with cardiac surgery; and (d) idiopathic (some of which may represent postural neuropathy). A less common cause is compression from a thyroid goitre or aortic aneurysm. Diaphragm elevation may also result from atelectasis, subphrenic abscess, hepatomegaly or subpulmonic effusion, and a similar radiographic pattern can also be produced by diaphragmatic eventration.
iii. A 'sniff test' done under fluoroscopy in the supine posture can aide in assessing the integrity of the phrenic nerve. The patient is asked to abruptly and strongly sniff while the diaphragm is observed. A paralysed diaphragm will paradoxically move up into the thorax as intrapleural pressure becomes more negative.

41 i. The lavage fluid shown is characteristic of pulmonary alveolar proteinosis, a disorder in which a phospholipid-rich proteinaceous material is deposited in the alveoli and bronchioles without associated lung fibrosis. Lung fluid obtained from whole lung lavage or BAL is milky in appearance and contains large macrophages with prominent cytoplasm.
ii. Whole lung lavage is the only treatment that is consistently successful. Often lavages of as much as 20 litres are performed at one session under general anaesthetic. The procedure is generally well tolerated and may be repeated as necessary, generally at 6- to 12-month intervals.
iii. Corticosteroids have not been shown to have a beneficial effect in this disorder and may be harmful. Inflammation does not appear to play a role in the pathogenesis. The condition is often self-limiting, with spontaneous remission after lavage clearance on radiography.

42 i. A hypopnoea.
ii. Apnoea is defined as complete cessation in airflow of 10 s or longer. Hypopnoea is more difficult to measure and is less precisely defined. Although there is wide agreement that hypopnoea occurs when there is a reduction in ventilation during sleep, opinion on how it is best measured and what degree of reduction is significant is very diverse. However, the reduction in ventilation must be accompanied by oxygen desaturation, arousal or both.

A decrease in ventilation can be documented directly by measurements of airflow and indirectly by measurements of thoraco- and/or abdominal movement. A wide range of devices which vary in both precision and reliability has been used to measure these parameters.

One definition of hypopnoea is a reduction of airflow of 50% or more, accompanied by a decrease in blood oxygen saturation of 4% or more. Another uses a 50% reduction in the thoracoabdominal movement as measured by inductive plethysmography.

43 The polysomnogram in **43** shows abnormal EMG traces, leg movement traces labelled LAT and RAT (left and right anterior tibial), together with an EEG recording (top six traces).

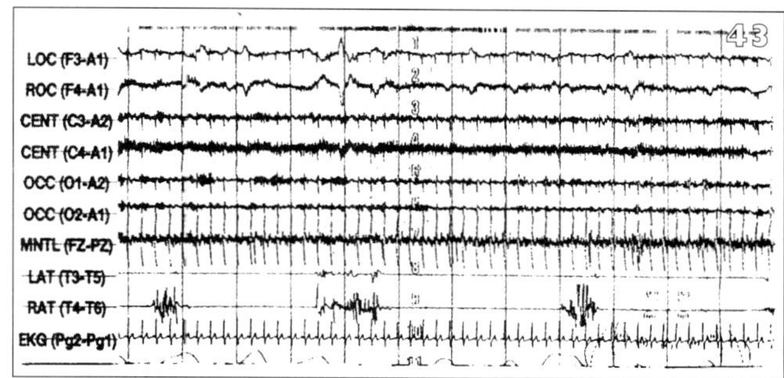

i. With what symptoms might this patient present?
ii. What is the relationship between this disorder, narcolepsy and/or obstructive sleep apnoea?

44 Intensive microbiological investigation of sputum, blood and bronchoalveolar lavage fluid (BAL) from the patient with this chest radiograph (**44**) has not detected a pathogen as a cause for his slowly progressive cough and dyspnoea. He is otherwise well with no evidence of extrapulmonary disease. The CD4 lymphocyte count is 0.2×10^9/l and the BAL showed abundant lymphocytes.

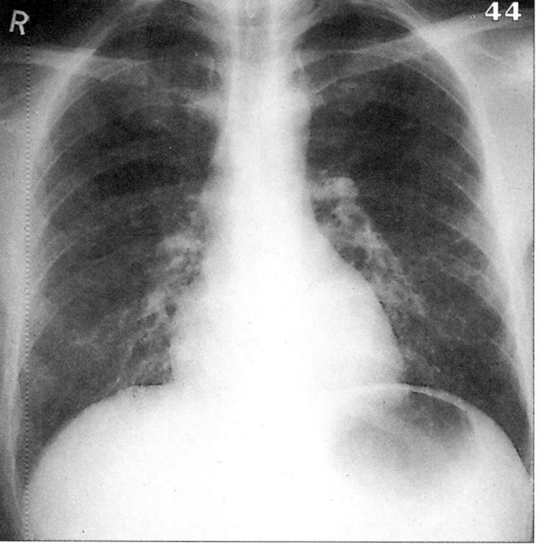

i. Name the possible causes for this illness.
ii. In the cases where opportunistic infection have been excluded as a cause, describe the usual setting for this illness.
iii. What would be your management of this patient?

45 A number of medications have been associated with the development of interstitial lung disease.
i. What pulmonary disorder is classically associated with nitrofurantoin?
ii. Name other medications associated with interstitial lung disease.

43 i. Periodic limb movement in sleep (PLMS) is a condition in which patients experience stereotyped repetitive movements once they are asleep. Patients can present with insomnia as there may be an irresistible urge to move the legs and excessive daytime somnolence. In addition, many patients with PLMS have restless leg syndrome (RLS) which manifests as discomfort in both legs accompanied by irresistible movements of the limbs during the day.

ii. PLMS can occur secondary to narcolepsy, central and obstructive sleep apnoea, and REM sleep behaviour disorder. It is more common in older patients, occurring in up to 30% of patients over 60 years old. Polysomnography with measurement of periodic leg movements by EMG is required to diagnose PLMS. Often period leg movements during drowsy wakefulness are seen, as in **43**. During sleep, leg movements are followed by an arousal. Treatment is primarily that of the underlying cause, or where none is apparent, hypnotics suppress the arousal.

44 i. Even when microbiological tests are negative, PCP would still be the most likely cause of this illness in an adult given the 5–10% rate of false-negative testing by microscopy of BAL. With appropriate testing it is less likely that cytomegalovirus infection would be missed. It is unlikely that rare causes such as pulmonary lymphoma or Kaposi's sarcoma are involved; therefore, it is likely that HIV-related lymphocytic interstitial pneumonitis (LIP) is the cause. This can be confirmed by open lung biopsy.

ii. LIP is very much more common in children and may account for 20–50% of paediatric AIDS.

iii. Such a patient should be treated with empirical anti-PCP therapy and there is also a valid argument for trying anti-CMV therapy. If this strategy fails, the next diagnostic option is an open lung biopsy. The cause of LIP is unknown but may represent an HIV-related immunological reaction. Treatment would be with anti-retroviral drugs and also steroids.

45 i. Both acute and chronic forms of drug-induced interstitial lung disease can occur in association with use of nitrofurantoin. The acute form begins within days (sometimes hours) of initiating therapy. Patients develop bilateral alveolar–interstitial infiltrates, fever, rigors and cough. Pleurisy may also occur. Symptoms resolve a few days after the drug has been stopped. The chronic form of disease can occur as long as 7 years after starting long-term antibiotic therapy and presents with an alveolitis and/or with interstitial fibrosis. Nitrofurantoin is the most common antibiotic associated with interstitial lung disease.

ii. Many additional medications are known to cause interstitial lung disease. The most common include various cytotoxic chemotherapeutic agents (e.g. bleomycin, cytoxan, methotrexate, nitrosoureas); and hydrochlorothiazide, gold and aspirin (acetylsalicylic acid). Other drugs causing pleural disease include bromocryptine, methysermide and methotrexate.

46 A 55-year-old man has had a large right pleural effusion (**46**) aspirated using a cannula on two occasions. Cytology has revealed malignant cells and he remains breathless. How would you proceed with the management of this patient?

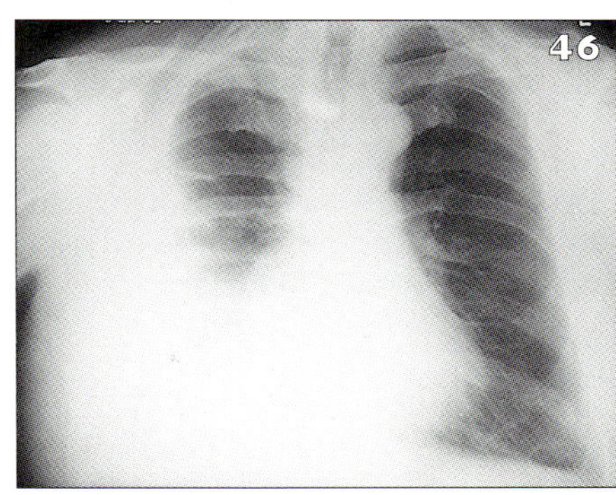

47 What device has been deployed in this patient's lower trachea (**47**)?

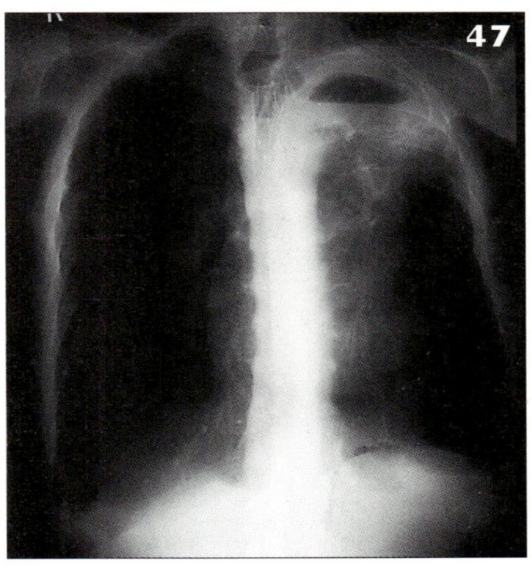

48 This chest radiograph (**48**) of a 58-year-old female ex-smoker presents with lethargy, a non-productive cough and mild generalized arthralgias. Her chest film shows bilateral hilar lymphadenopathy and an abdominal CT showed paraortic lymph nodes. Her serum ACE, biochemical profile and full blood count was normal, but her ESR was 80 mm/h
i. What is the differential diagnosis?
ii. What other investigations would you do?

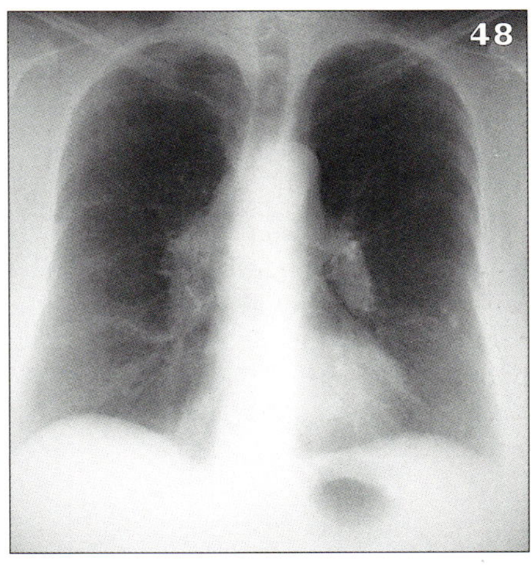

46 He clearly has a sizeable and recurrent right-sided pleural effusion with an underlying malignant process. Management is directed towards palliation of his symptoms which include breathlessness. Thoracoscopy should be undertaken if he is fit enough for a general anaesthetic. The extent of his pleural disease can then be assessed and the pleural cavity drained to dryness. Then if the lung is able to expand fully, pleurodesis should be effected by the insufflation of sterile talc into the pleural cavity. Alternatively, a chest drain can be inserted under local anaesthetic and once the pleural effusion has completely drained, a talc suspension can be introduced into the pleural cavity via the drain. The chest radiograph performed after chest drain insertion in this case showed the lung had not re-expanded. Therefore, pleurodesis cannot be performed as the pleural surfaces are not apposed. In this situation palliation can be effected by the introduction of a pleuro-peritoneal shunt. This allows the patient to drain the pleural effusion into the abdomen through a manually operated one-way valve sited under the skin of the lower chest wall.

47 An expandable metal stent. The patient's lower trachea was narrowed by extrinsic compression due to a tumour. Stents are used to palliate breathlessness due to extrinsic compression of major airways. They are deployed under general anaesthetic with the use of a rigid bronchoscope. Laser resection may precede placement if there is additional endoluminal disease. Problems with this type of airway stent include the fact that they cannot be removed, ingrowth of tumour between the wires, and long-term penetration of the bronchial wall with possible stent fracture. None of these problems occur with silastic stents, which are flexible and remain in place due to small protuberances on their outer surface.

Patients with stents must regularly check peak flows to monitor for the effect of blockage of the stent by secretions or tumour ingrowth, although obstruction may be quite severe before peak flows start to fall. They should also have 3-monthly check bronchoscopies to look for these complications. With silastic stents sudden development of cough or breathlessness may indicate stent migration has occurred.

48 i. A normal serum ACE does not rule out sarcoidosis. A very high ESR is not common in sarcoidosis and although para-aortic lymphadenopathy may occur in sarcoidosis, metastatic carcinoma and lymphoma must be excluded.
ii. Although a transbronchial biopsy may be useful in a younger patient, a mediastinoscopy is more likely to obtain a diagnosis here. Her mediastinal lymph nodes showed adenocarcinoma and no primary was found. Sometimes mediastinal lymphoma may be misdiagnosed as sarcoidosis if there is no biopsy confirmation and even with a lymph node biopsy misdiagnosis can occur as regional lymph nodes draining carcinomas and lymphomas can show granulomatous reactions which mimic sarcoidosis. An elevated serum ACE occasionally occurs in Hodgkin's disease and non-Hodgkin's lymphomas – especially histiocytic lymphomas – and may lead to misdiagnosis.

49 These lung function results (Table) are from a 40-year-old woman 18 months post-allogeneic bone marrow transplantation (BMT) for acute myeloid leukaemia. There was no acute change in the results after bronchodilator. She had developed skin and gastrointestinal graft-versus-host disease at 12 months post-BMT.

i. What is the likely cause of the lung function abnormalities?
ii. What are the common pulmonary complications of bone marrow transplantation?

Test	Predicted	Range	Result	% predicted
PEFR (l/min)	374	318–430	122	33
FEV$_1$ (l)	2.31	1.96–2.65	0.85	37
FVC (l)	3.04	2.58–3.49	1.84	61
FEV (%)	75	64–86	46	62
DL$_{CO}$ (mmol/min/kPa)*	7.61	6.47–8.75	5.90	78
VA (l)	–	–	3.05	–
K$_{CO}$ mmol/min/kPa/l)**	1.70	1.44–1.95	1.94	114

*DL$_{CO}$ = transfer factor. **K$_{CO}$ = transfer coefficient, i.e. DL$_{CO}$/VA.

50 A 40-year-old man presented with marked lethargy, cough, polyuria and thirst and this skin lesion on his elbow. His serum ACE is markedly elevated.
i. What is the skin lesion (50)?
ii. What is the cause of his polyuria and thirst?
iii. What is the role of serum ACE in the management of sarcoidosis?

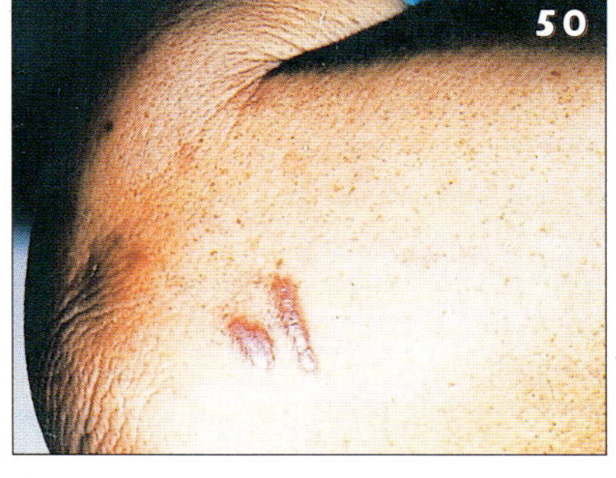

51 i. This 30-year-old man complained of a chronic cough for 3 months. His chest radiograph was normal.
i. Interpret the lung function test (Table).
ii. What is the diagnosis?

Test	Predicted	Range	Result	% predicted
PEFR (l/min)	531	451–611	344	65
FEV$_1$ (l)	3.16	2.69–3.63	1.78	56
FVC (l)	4.03	3.43–4.65	3.02	75
FEV$_1$/FVC (%)	71	61–82	58	83

Post-bronchodilator			
Test	Predicted	Range	Result
PEFR (l/min)	–	–	430
FEV$_1$ (l)	–	–	2.22
FVC (l)	–	–	3.10
FEV$_1$/FVC (%)	–	–	71

49 i. There is severe airflow obstruction. The likely cause is bronchiolitis obliterans, a progressive irreversible fibrosis of small airways. It may stabilize, leaving the patient with severe breathlessness or, in a significant number, it may be fatal. Treatment with immunosuppressive drugs may slow the rate of progression but increases the risk of opportunistic infection. Risks for the development of the condition include chronic graft-versus-host disease, and episodes of preceding pulmonary toxicity.

ii. Idiopathic interstitial pneumonitis is well described occurring at approximately 1–2 months post-transplant and is almost always fatal. This may be a drug toxicity effect of the common agents used for pre-transplant chemotherapy (conditioning), Busulfan and cyclophosphamide. CMV pneumonitis may occur later and may be diagnosed by transbronchial biopsy, where the hallmark is large cells with nuclei containing large basophilic inclusions and or with fluorescent antibody testing of bronchoalveolar lavage fluid. It also is invariably fatal. Bacterial and fungal pneumonias also occur. A less common fatal complication is pulmonary haemorrhage.

50 i. The skin lesion is cutaneous sarcoidosis which looks like keloid.

ii. His polyuria and thirst are from hypercalcaemia. His 24-hour urine calcium shows marked hypercalciuria also caused by the overproduction of calcitriol by sarcoid granulomas and pulmonary macrophages. He should be rehydrated and commenced on high-dose prednisolone.

iii. World-wide an elevated serum ACE has a sensitivity of 57% with a specificity of 90%, a positive predictive value of 90% and a negative predictive of 60%. The serum elevation in sarcoidosis is due to the epithelioid cells of sarcoid granulomas and pulmonary macrophages. It is elevated also in silicosis, severe diabetes, hyperthyroidism and cirrhosis and is always markedly elevated in Gaucher's disease. ACE inhibitors used in cardiac failure and hypertension markedly depress serum ACE. Serum ACE is more likely to be elevated in severe active sarcoidosis especially with hypercalcaemia and falls as the disease remits or is treated with corticosteroids. It is an invaluable test for the long-term monitoring of disease activity.

51 i. A 25% improvement in FEV_1 following bronchodilator therapy. A difference of more than 12% between two efforts at spirometry is considered significant. The greater the improvement after inhaled bronchodilator and the faster the spirometry returns to normal, the more likely is the diagnosis to be asthma. Some patients with chronic obstructive airways disease will show improvement in spirometry, usually after large doses of bronchodilator. An acute change may not be seen in asthmatics if they have been taking regular bronchodilators before testing or if their treatment is optimal with inhaled corticosteroids, thus stabilizing their condition, or with severe or persistent asthma.

ii. Bronchial asthma. (Marked post-bronchodilator changes such as these indicate poor control of asthma in patients who are already on treatment.)

52 This chest radiograph (52) in a
36-year-old male smoker who
presented for a routine life insurance
medical examination. He is in good
health with a normal physical
examination.
i. What is the provisional diagnosis?
ii. What radiographic stage is the
disease?
iii. What investigations would you
suggest to confirm the likely
diagnosis?

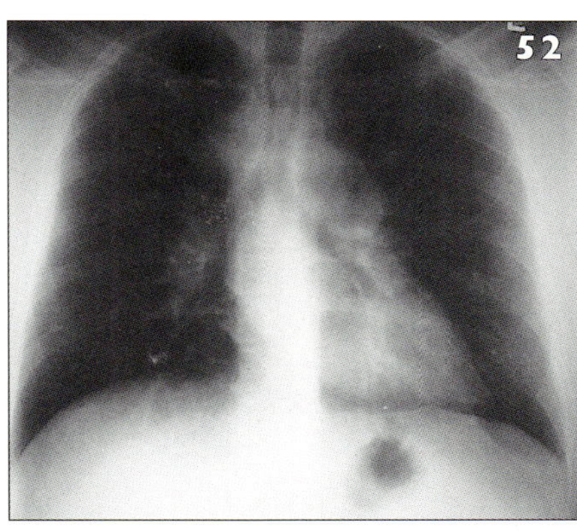

53 Shown is the chest radiograph (53) of a 61-year-old man with symptoms
of high fever, headache, cough and
pleuritic chest pain of 3 days'
duration. He smoked cigarettes,
drank 40 units of alcohol a week and
took prednisone on alternate days for
rheumatoid arthritis. He appeared
obtunded and tachypnoeic and was
hypotensive. A Gram stain of sputum
obtained by nasotracheal suction
showed many polymorphonuclear
leukocytes but no apparent bacteria.
i. What are the radiographic findings?
ii. What is the most likely diagnosis?
iii. What is the most appropriate
treatment?

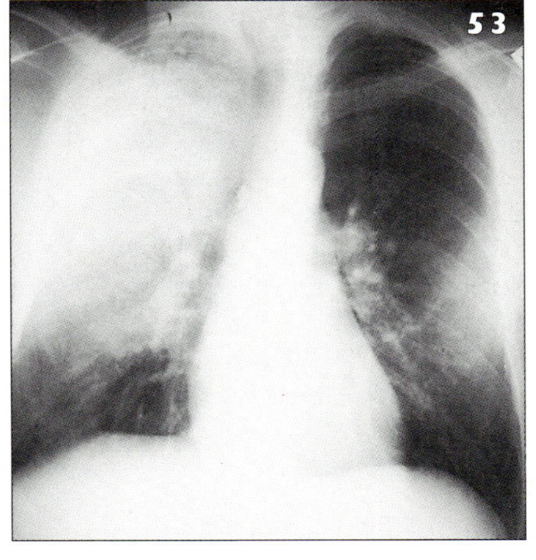

54 This woman of 58 has had
similar appearances on her chest
radiograph (54) for over 5 years. She
does not have significant respiratory
symptoms. What is the differential
diagnosis?

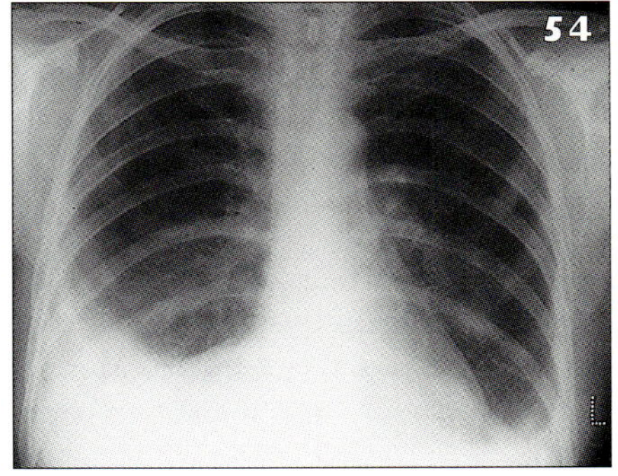

52 i. Sarcoidosis is the most likely diagnosis in a fit young male, although it is less common in smokers.
ii. This patient has stage I disease. Sarcoidosis is staged as follows: normal chest radiograph, stage 0; bilateral hilar adenopathy, stage I; bilateral hilar adenopathy and parenchymal infiltrates, stage II; parenchymal disease only, stage III; and irreversible pulmonary fibrosis and/or bulla formation, stage IV. Stage I disease occurs in about 50% of patients. A diffuse reticulonodular pattern is the most common parenchymal abnormality. Involvement of the anterior mediastinal lymph nodes and unilateral hilar lymphadenopathy is less common in sarcoidosis and raises the possibility of lymphoma or malignancy.
iii. A markedly elevated serum angiotensin-converting enzyme (ACE) alone may be sufficient in patients with classic clinical features. It is sometimes advisable if the presentation is unusual to obtain histological confirmation by fibre-optic transbronchial lung biopsy or mediastinoscopy to exclude other possibilities. Serum calcium and a 24-hour urine calcium are recommended to identify unsuspected hypercalciuria or hypercalcaemia.

53 i. There is dense consolidation of the right upper lobe with prominent air bronchograms.
ii. This patient has a severe community-acquired pneumonia which is most often caused by *Str. pneumoniae*, *Staph. aureus* or Gram-negative bacilli including *Legionella* sp. In this setting, a Gram stain demonstrating a purulent exudate but no organisms is highly suggestive of *Legionella* infection. Legionellae are facultative, intracellular pathogens which infect alveolar macrophages and cause a pneumonic illness which is often accompanied by systemic manifestations which can be severe. Corticosteroid-treated patients, cigarette smokers and heavy drinkers are particularly susceptible. The organisms are poorly seen on Gram-stains of sputa but can some-times be visualized using basic fuchsin-based stains or direct fluorescent antibodies. Isolation requires special culture medium and several days of incubation. Serological testing can confirm infection after the fact but cannot guide antibiotic therapy.
iii. Treatment with erythromycin for 3 weeks is recommended. Rifampicin should be added in severe cases and an attempt should be made to minimize corticosteroid use.

54 The chest radiograph (54) shows moderate bilateral pleural effusions. The absence of cardiac enlargement and significant dyspnoea should exclude left ventricular failure (LVF) although cardiac failure can occur with a normal cardiac silhouette in patients with mitral stenosis or constrictive pericarditis. It is most likely that she has an inflammatory pleurisy, probably due to autoimmune disease such as systemic lupus erythematosis or rheumatoid arthritis. The patient shown here suffered from chronic rheumatoid arthritis. Other possible causes include vasculitides such as polyarteritis nodosa, Wegener's granulomatosis and, polyserositis, drug reactions, e.g. hydralazine, phenytoin, phenothiazines and practolol, lymphatic hypoplasia (yellow nail syndrome) and hypothyroidism. In general, bilateral effusions suggest a systemic cause and unilateral fluid a local cause.

55 A previously well patient presents with mild, gradual-onset left pleuritic pain. The lung scan [55 – KR, krypton (ventilation) image; TC, technetium (perfusion) image] is reported as showing intermediate probability for pulmonary embolism (PE). How would you proceed?

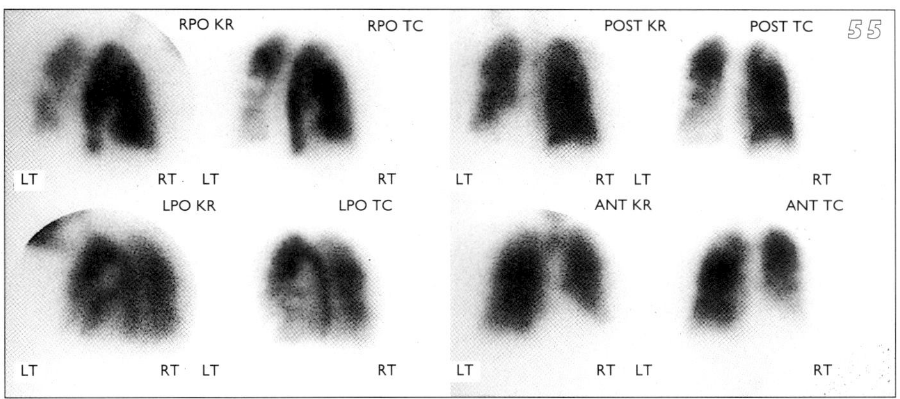

56 This 16-year-old girl presented with myasthenic symptoms and underwent routine evaluation for thymectomy which included a normal plain chest radiograph.
i. What abnormality was found on the CT scan (56)?
ii. What are the usual characteristics of the thymus in myasthenia patients?
iii. What treatment should be advised? What is the significance of the lesion present?

57 i. What is the likely cause of this (57) gastrointestinal complication in a CF patient?
ii. What is the best treatment.

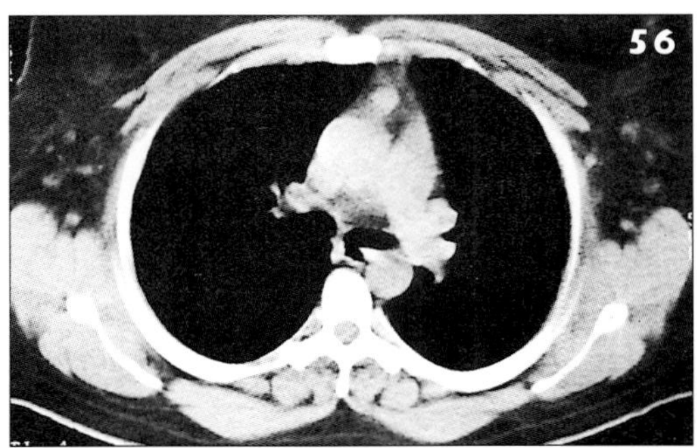

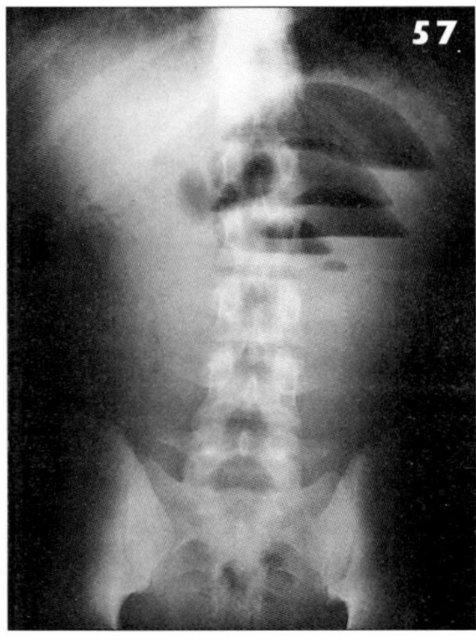

55 Based on PIOPED criteria, intermediate probability scans had a likelihood of pulmonary embolism (based on pulmonary angiogram) of between 16–66%. On the other hand, high-probability scans with high clinical probability have a 96% chance of having PTE and normal scans even with high clinical probability effectively rule out PTE. Therefore, intermediate and low probability scans can be regarded as being of indeterminate probability and patients require further investigation. Papers published subsequent to the PIOPED study include tables derived by including both moderate and large-sized perfusion defects which further improves the specificity of ventilation perfusion scanning. The PIOPED data were calculated using only large segmental defects. A Doppler ultrasound of leg vein, or venography should be performed. The clinical probability here is low and if no leg vein thrombosis is demonstrated no further investigation is necessary. If the clinical probability is uncertain or high and leg vein investigations are negative, then pulmonary angiography should be performed, preferably within 72 hours of the onset of symptoms.

56 i. A small (2 cm) thymoma can be seen in the retrosternal space.
ii. Most myasthenia cases (90%) occur after puberty. Thymoma is present in only 10–15% of these adult cases and is exceptionally uncommon in juvenile onset cases. Approximately 10–25% of adult cases have a normal gland but the majority exhibit lymphoid follicular hyperplasia.
iii. It is usual to recommend thymectomy for all cases of myasthenia except those which are very mild or confined to the occulomotor muscles. It should be performed in all patients with a thymoma.

The available data regarding outcome are confused as more severe cases proceed to surgery whereas less severe cases are managed by anticholinesterase medication. Thymectomy appears to be associated with better long-term survival and clinical result than medical therapy. For those with hyperplasia, 15% are drug free following surgery, 25% are in drug-maintained remission, 50% are clinically improved and 10% are unchanged. The presence of a thymoma is associated with a significantly poorer result from surgery.

57 i. The radiograph in **57** illustrates the typical features of the **distal intestinal obstruction syndrome** (DIOS) with dilated loops of small bowel. It is due to inspissated intestinal contents in the distal ileum and proximal colon.

The more common causes are insufficient prescription of pancreatic enzymes or patient non-compliance with enzyme treatment.
ii. Treatment of the acute event involves rehydration and the administration of oral gastrograffin (100 ml in 400 ml of water in older patients). It may also be given as an enema. For resistant cases, large volumes (5–6 l) of a balanced electrolyte intestinal lavage solution administered by a nasogastric tube is very effective.

Surgical treatment should be avoided.

58 A patient with severe, stable
COPD has stopped smoking and
bronchodilator therapy has been
optimized (58). He continues to be
dyspnoeic. Corticosteroid therapy is
now considered.
i. When should corticosteroids be
used in the long-term management of
COPD?
ii. How should a steroid trial be conducted in
stable patients with COPD?

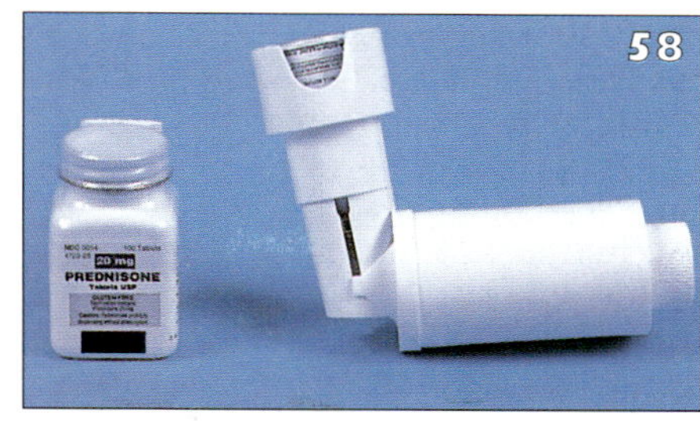

59 The cytology specimen
in (59) was obtained by
fine-needle aspiration of a
peripheral mass seen on
chest radiograph. What
does it show and how
accurate is this procedure
in predicting the histology
of masses removed by
surgery?

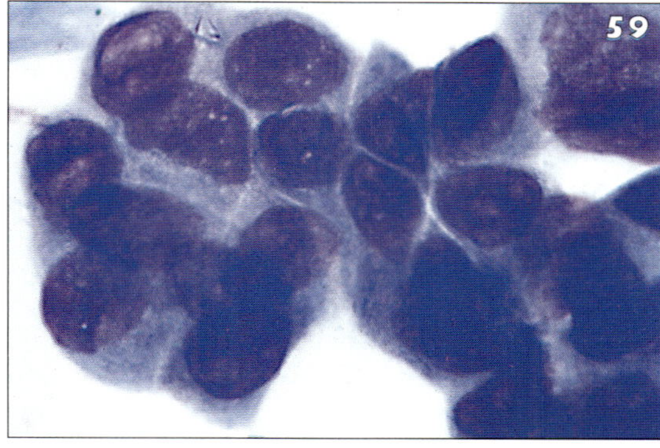

60 i. Describe the appearances in
this chest radiograph (60).
ii. What are the likely causative
organisms?
iii. What are the causes of a swollen
lobe in the presence of pneumonia?

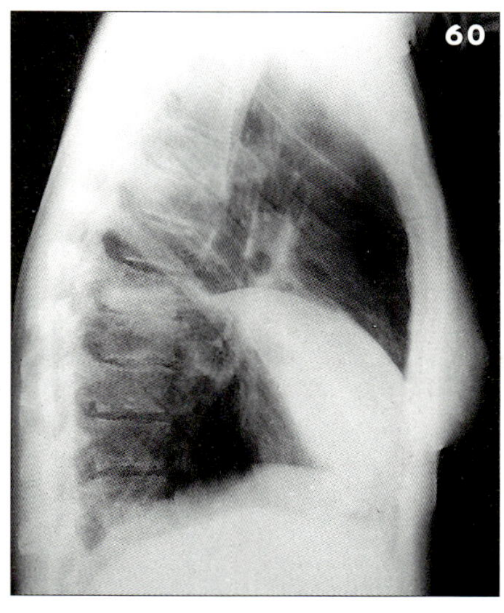

58 i. The place of corticosteroids in the long-term management of COPD remains controversial. However, in the individual patient who remains symptomatic despite anticholinergic and β_2 agonist inhalers and oral theophylline, an 'n of 1' steroid trial should be performed.

ii. The effect of corticosteroids should be assessed by spirometry (with and without bronchodilators) obtained before and after the steroid trial. Most recommend starting systemic corticosteroids (e.g. prednisone at approximately 0.5 mg/kg daily, or equivalent) for 2–3 weeks. An improvement in the FEV_1 of at least 20% and an absolute increase of at least 0.2 l are regarded as evidence of steroid responsiveness (>30% improvement is required by some experts). If a response is observed the steroids are then tapered to the lowest effective dose and/or the patient should be switched to inhaled steroids. It may be that a small improvement in lung function is outweighed by corticosteroid side effects. In those who are not steroid-responsive, the steroid should be tapered and discontinued over approximately 1 week.

59 This shows non-small-cell carcinoma. The features are not specific enough to differentiate between squamous cell carcinoma and adenocarcinoma; however, they do show large hyperchromatic cells with abundant cytoplasm and nuclear atypia. When removed surgically the final histology may be squamous cell or adenocarcinoma, or if no specific features are shown it may be termed large cell carcinoma, a diagnosis of exclusion. Cytologically, small cell carcinoma shows cells with minimal cytoplasm and uniformly hyperchromatic and moulded nuclei. They are not always truly small on smears and nuclear changes are not constant. Also there may be a number of cell types expressed to varying degrees within a single tumour since all lung tumours most likely arise from a single stem cell rather than from cells which have already differentiated into for example squamous cells. In general, cytological samples obtained by fine-needle aspiration are able to distinguish small-cell from non-small-cell lung cases very accurately – but are cell type-specific in up to 70% of non-small-cell carcinomas.

60 i. This lateral chest radiograph (60) shows homogeneous consolidation within the middle lobe. The horizontal fissure is bowed upwards, suggesting some swelling of the lobe.

ii. *Str. pneumoniae* is the most common cause of community-acquired pneumonia and is the most typical cause of lobar pneumonia. However, it is often unappreciated that most other common bacterial causes of pneumonia can also cause lobar consolidation including legionella, *Staph. aureus* and as many as 50% of *Myc. pneumoniae* pneumonias are lobar.

iii. *K. pneumoniae* is also a cause of a swollen lobe on the chest radiograph but as in this example, which is due to *Myc. pneumoniae*, any bacterial pathogen can potentially do this.

61 The mediastinum may be divided into three compartments for classification of mass lesions: anterior, visceral and paravertebral (**61**). The anterior compartment lies between the sternum and the anterior surface of the pericardium and the great vessels which forms the anterior border of the visceral compartment. This contains the intrathoracic organs and therefore extends posteriorly to the vertebral column. The paravertebral compartment comprises the paravertebral spaces. List the more common lesions found in each compartment.

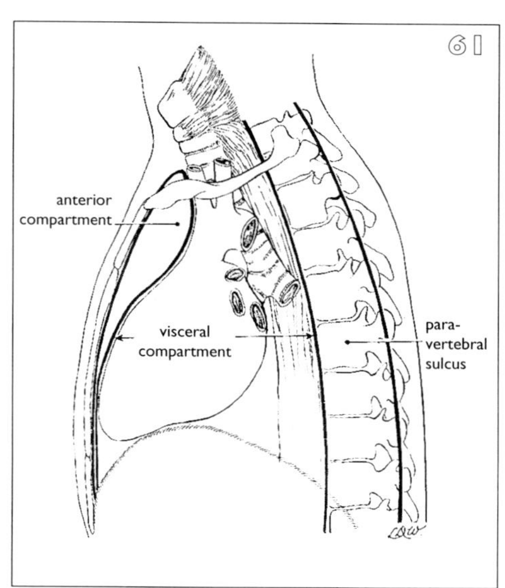

62 The abnormalities seen in the chest radiograph (**62**) developed suddenly in a patient with history of recent intravenous drug use.
i. What is the differential diagnosis?
ii. How might information obtained from the pulmonary artery catheter affect the differential diagnosis?
iii. How might the history of heroin use relate to the abnormalities shown?

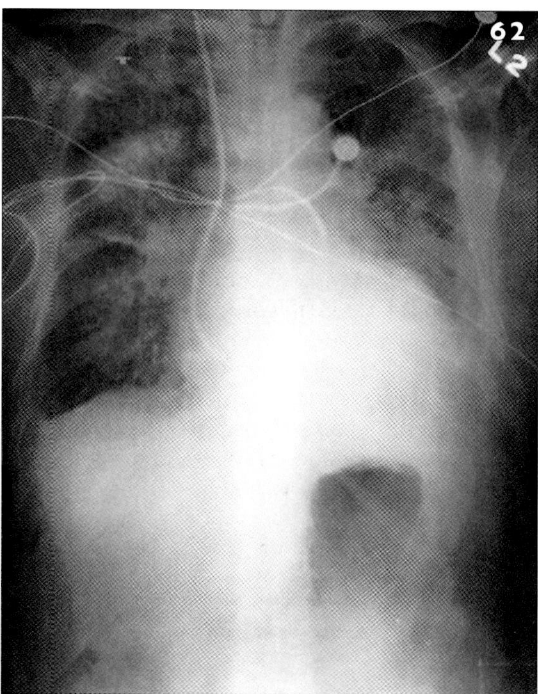

61 Clearly, any tissue element may give rise to a tumour so that rarities such as sarcomas are possible but the more common lesions are :
- Anterior: lymphoma, thymoma, thymic hyperplasia, germ cell tumours (teratomas, dermoid cysts, malignant germ cell tumours).
- Visceral: secondary mediastinal tumour, lymphoma, retrosternal thyroid, aortic aneurysm, hiatus hernia, lymphadenopathy, enterogenous cyst, bronchogenic cyst, pleuropericardial cyst, ganglionoma.
- Posterior: neurogenic tumour, lymphoma, haemangioma.

Note that the older classification of superior, anterior, middle and posterior mediastinum may be encountered. This can be confusing as it utilizes arbitrary boundaries between these areas. The superior mediastinum lies above a line drawn from T4 to the manubrial–sternal junction and thus includes elements of the three compartments described above. Similarly, the posterior mediastinum includes both the paravertebral compartment and that portion of the visceral compartment which lies behind the trachea and heart. This older classification leads to the same lesion potentially appearing under several descriptive areas. For example, a moderate retrosternal thyroid would be a superior mediastinal lesion which might easily extend through the middle mediastinum into the retrotracheal section of the posterior mediastinum. The compartment classification would place this lesion entirely in the visceral compartment.

62 i. The differential diagnosis of acute interstitial infiltrates can be divided into cardiogenic causes and conditions resulting in increased vascular permeability. Cardiogenic causes include congestive heart failure, myocardial infarction or coronary insufficiency, acute valvular heart disease, severe volume overload and acute diastolic dysfunction. Increased permeability can result from near drowning, heroin or other drug overdose, sepsis, chest trauma, burns or exposure to toxic gases. The oedema that develops at high altitude may result from abnormalities in both intravascular pressure and permeability.
ii. A pulmonary artery catheter allows measurement of the pulmonary arterial occlusion (wedge) pressure as a reflection of the left ventricular preload and/or the intravascular hydrostatic pressure in the pulmonary capillaries (ignoring the effects of possible venoconstriction) and can frequently separate cardiac from permeability problems. A wedge pressure of >18 cm H_2O suggests cardiac abnormalities.
iii. As stated above, heroin and other opiate drugs – illicit as well as conventional use – can cause acute non-cardiogenic pulmonary oedema. Intravenous drugs are also associated with alterations in consciousness leading to widespread aspiration, to acute myocardial dysfunction (cocaine) or to valvular incompetence (acute bacterial endocarditis).

63 This middle-aged male patient complained of mild dysphagia. A barium examination and endoscopy both showed only smooth mild extrinsic compression of the oesophagus. A CT scan was obtained (**63**).
i. What abnormality is present?
ii. What is the differential diagnosis?
iii. How may this be treated?

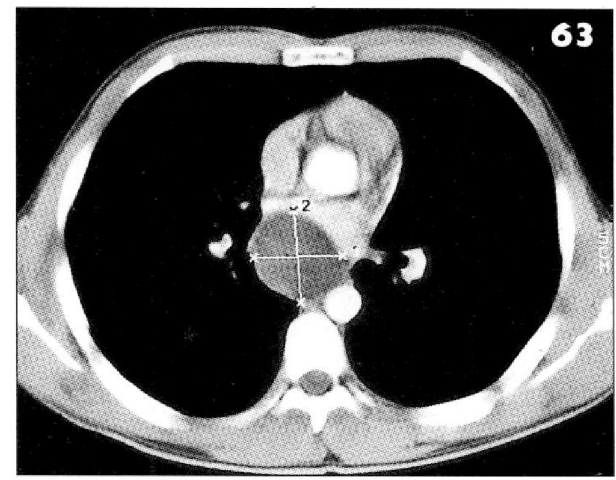

64 A 60-year-old female patient underwent major abdominal surgery for a non-malignant condition; she spent some days on the intensive care unit. Her chest radiograph at follow-up, some weeks later, showed a wide mediastinum; the subsequent CT scan is shown here (**64**).
i. What is the abnormality?
ii. What is the likely cause and how would you further investigate the patient?

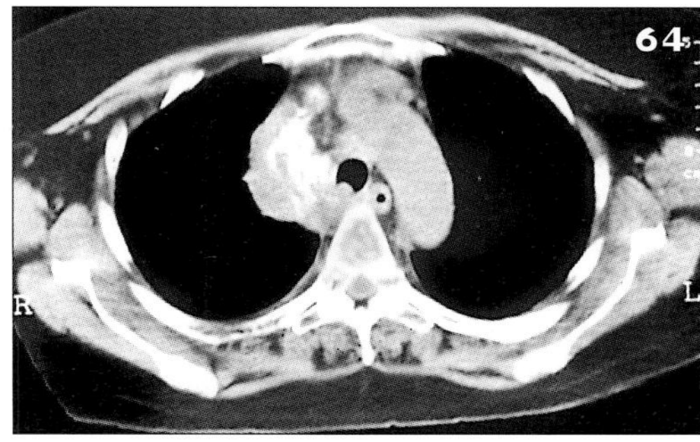

65 Shown (**65**) is a CT scan from a 75-year-old Chinese man who has chronic sputum production which has not increased over the past 4 years. Sputum cultures have grown *Mycobacterium intracellulare*.
i. Should antituberculous chemotherapy be given?
ii. Should isolation procedures be used?

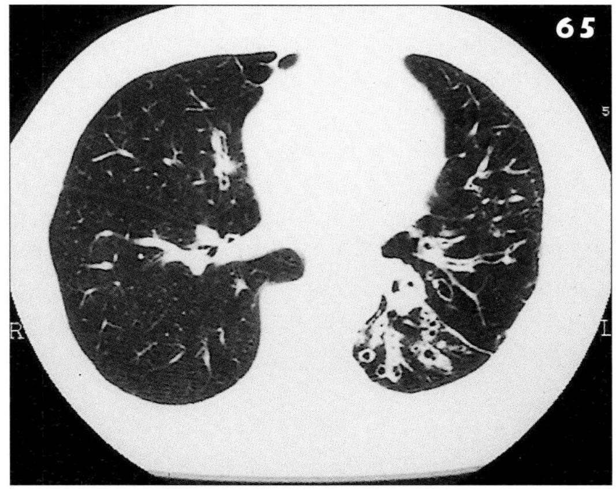

63 i. The lesion is a smooth-walled cyst in the visceral compartment.

ii. This is most likely a foregut cyst. During the development of the tracheobronchial tree from the foregut, cells may be sequestered which subsequently give rise to foregut cysts, i.e. a bronchogenic or enterogenous cyst. It is not possible to say accurately without histological examination of the lining epithelium and even then the features may be non-specific.

In a child other possibilities would exist. A neurenteric cyst connects with the meninges and is normally found in young children with associated spinal deformities. These occasionally also communicate with the gastrointestinal tract. A gastroenteric cyst is lined by gastric mucosa and may communicate with the stomach below the diaphragm. It is also normally encountered in children and associated with spinal abnormalities.

iii. Opinion varies regarding best management of foregut cysts. Small cysts which are asymptomatic chance findings can be observed but if bronchial or oesophageal compression symptoms are present they should be removed or marsupialized to the pleural cavity.

64 i. The CT scan (**64**) shows a mediastinal mass in the right paratracheal region.

ii. This could indicate mediastinal lymphadenopathy but the patient is likely to have had a radiograph before her abdominal surgery. Was this normal? If it was, taking into consideration that the patient spent time on the ITU, were any central lines inserted in the perioperative period? If internal jugular lines were used then it is likely that the apparent mass on the current CT scan represents haematoma and follow-up with plain chest radiography is indicated. If doubt remains as to the aetiology of the 'mass' then the investigation of choice would be mediastinoscopy.

65 i. This organism – which is ubiquitous in the environment – is usually regarded as a colonizer of damaged airways, such as the extensive area of bronchiectasis depicted in the CT scan. This patient's plain chest radiograph had features of previous tuberculous infection which may have been the cause of the bronchiectasis.

Clinically a typical mycobacteria, of which *M. intracellulare* is one, can cause disease indistinguishable from typical *M. tuberculosis* infection. Along with the other opportunistic mycobacterial organisms it may also arise in patients with altered immune function.

ii. The decision to treat would be based on isolating the organism in at least two sputum samples (as it may be a contaminant) and the presence of radiograph abnormalities consistent with tuberculosis, particularly where those abnormalities are progressive. The decision to embark on treatment should include consideration that the length of treatment will be 2 years, that the response rates to therapy may be as low as 50%, and that the most effective drug regimen is yet to be determined.

66 An elderly patient with severe COPD has the following room air, arterial blood gas tensions when breathing room air: pH, 7.38; $PaCO_2$, 46 mmHg (6.0 kPa); PaO_2, 54 mmHg (7.1 kPa).

i. Is supplemental oxygen (**66**) appropriate for this patient?
ii. If oxygen is to be prescribed, for how many hours a day should it be used?
iii. What are the benefits of long-term oxygen therapy?

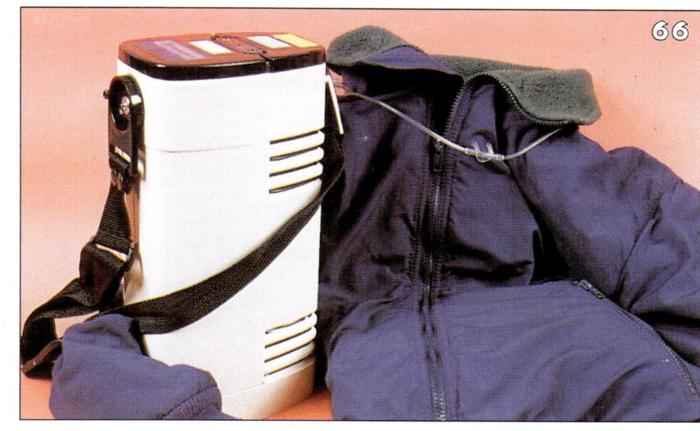

67 i. What is the allergen likely to be present in high concentrations in this living environment (**67**)?
ii. How can environmental control be achieved?
iii. What is the role of immunotherapy in this type of allergy?

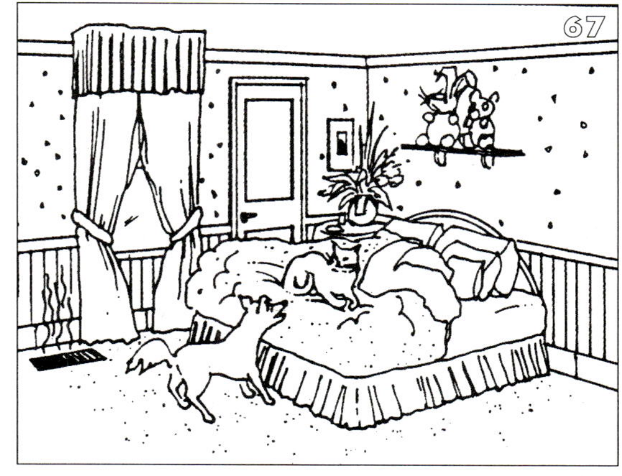

68 Organ transplantation is the optimum management for preterminal disease in CF.
i. What is the current survival?
ii. When should a patient be referred for transplantation consideration?

66 i. Yes. Indications for long-term oxygen therapy include: (a) resting room air PaO_2 <55 mmHg (7.3 kPa) or O_2 saturation <88%; (b) resting room air PaO_2 56–59 mmHg (7.3–8.0 kPa) or O_2 saturation 89% plus evidence of end-organ dysfunction due to chronic hypoxia [e.g. P-pulmonale on the ECG (P waves >3 mm in II, III, aVF), right heart failure (pedal oedema), erythrocythaemia (haematocrit >55%)].
ii. Continuous, 15–24 hours per day. The improvement in survival with long-term oxygen therapy is proportional to the number of hours per day the O_2 is used. The NOTT study in 1981 showed improved 2-year survival in patients having nasal oxygen continuously, compared with 12 hours per day (40.8% versus 22%). Similar improvements were shown in the MRC study 1981 where 5-year mortality in COPD patients receiving 2 l nasal oxygen for 15 hours per day was 45.2% compared with 66.7% in non recipients of O_2.
iii. Long-term oxygen therapy improves survival, pulmonary haemodynamics, exercise capacity, and neuropsychological performance in patients with COPD.

67 i. House dust mites thrive in the environment pictured. The allergens involved include the *Dermatophagoides* species of mite (*D. pteronyssinus, D. farinae, D. microceras*). *D. pteronyssinus* has four allergens, I–IV. Development of atopy to the mite is genetically linked. If one parent is allergic there is a 50% chance that the child will be allergic; if both parents are allergic the chance is 80%. The intensity and duration of exposure in early childhood correlates with subsequent sensitization.
ii. The mites live and die in bedding, carpeting, curtains and upholstered furniture. Central heating and limited ventilation also predispose to mite build-up. Aggressive reduction of mite numbers can be accomplished by:
- Washing the bedding at >55°C at least weekly.
- Vacuuming the carpets.
- Replacing the carpets with vinyl or hardwood floors.
- Keeping the relative humidity <50% with air conditioning.
- Enclosing the mattress in a vinyl cover.

iii. Immunotherapy involves the administration of increasing amounts of allergenic extracts with the idea of reducing clinical reactivity. It works in a small number of patients. A very small risk of death due to anaphylaxis with this treatment should always be discussed first.

68 i. Survival following transplantation depends upon the fitness of the patient at transplantation. In two UK transplant units actuarial survival for 111 patients at 1 year was 69–72% and at 2 years was 57–58%. It is crucial that the procedure is performed in centres expert in lung transplantation in CF patients.

69 This chest radiograph (**69**) is of a 26-year-old man who had repeated syncopal episodes and required permanent pacemaker insertion for complete heart block. He also had experienced several months of lethargy and intermittent dull retrosternal chest pain.
i. What diagnostic possibility does the radiograph show?
ii. What investigations would you suggest?
iii. What is the cause of the pain?
iv. When are corticosterioids indicated?

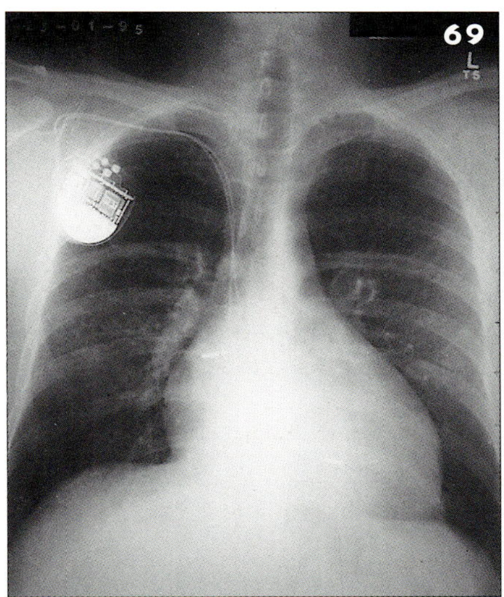

70 i. How is the maximum exercise ventilation predicted in patients with chronic airflow obstruction?
ii. Ventilation for a given oxygen uptake is often excessive in patients with airflow obstruction. What factors contribute to an excessively high ventilation during exercise in these patients and others with pulmonary disease?

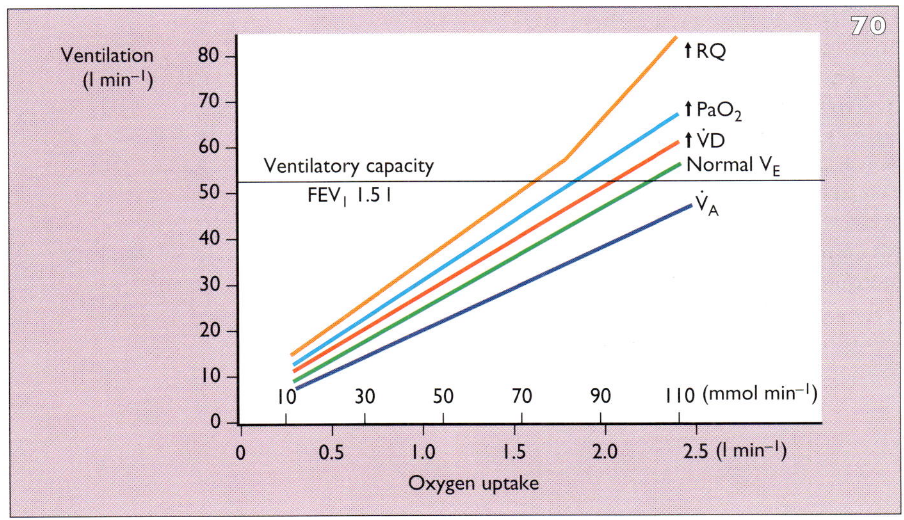

69 i. This patient has stage III sarcoidosis with cardiac involvement. Cardiac disease in this condition may cause a range of ventricular and supraventricular arrhythmias and conduction defects. Cardiomyopathy may develop rarely.

ii. ECG and Holter monitoring to document arrhythmias; 2D echocardiography may show ventricular septal thinning, localized regional wall abnormalities or a generalized cardiomyopathy. Thallium scintigraphy may show regions of abnormal perfusion. Endocardial biopsy may yield positive histology in less than 40% of cases.

iii. Chest pain in sarcoidosis is common (at least 25%) and may be pleuritic or dull and retrosternal. It may be severe and sometimes mimic a myocardial infarct. Cardiac sarcoidosis is a difficult diagnosis to establish without a myocardial biopsy. Even then, a clear association with an arrhythmia and sarcoidosis is difficult unless the sarcoidosis is clearly active in other sites.

iv. Arrhythmias and cardiomyopathy should be treated in the usual way. Corticosteroids would be indicated if standard treatment was ineffective or if the sarcoidosis was active at other sites. Monitoring of the response of cardiac sarcoid to corticosteroids is difficult.

70 i. The maximum exercise ventilation is predicted as the $FEV_1 \times 35$ in litres.

ii. The ventilatory response to exercise is linear until anaerobic metabolism stimulates ventilation further by a decrease in the pH.

Minute ventilation is a combination of alveolar ventilation and dead space ventilation. In patients with airflow obstruction, the contribution from the dead space (VD), both anatomical and physiological, increases. The worse the airflow obstruction, the higher the minute ventilation has to be in order to maintain a normal rate of gas exchange.

Other factors that will increase minute ventilation are:

- Hypoxia – this will add to ventilatory drive and ventilation will rise.
- Respiratory exchange ratio (RQ) – if the patient makes an anaerobic contribution to exercise, either due to an abnormal diet, e.g. high fat, low carbohydrate, or because the anaerobic mechanisms 'kick in' early due to poor aerobic metabolism.

70 shows an idealized scheme where minute ventilation comprises alveolar ventilation, dead space ventilation (VD) and contributions due to hypoxia (PaO_2) and an increase in respiratory exchange ratio (RQ). The horizontal line shows the predicted maximum exercise ventilation for an FEV_1 of 1.5 l and it can be seen as the various factors cause the minute ventilation to rise, the curves will move to the left, limiting exercise prematurely.

71 This man was treated with six courses of cytotoxic chemotherapy for small-cell lung cancer 18 months ago. He returned to the clinic feeling well, but had noticed some lesions in his neck.
i. What is illustrated in 71?
ii. How should this be treated?
iii. What is the value of chemotherapy in relapsed small-cell lung cancer?

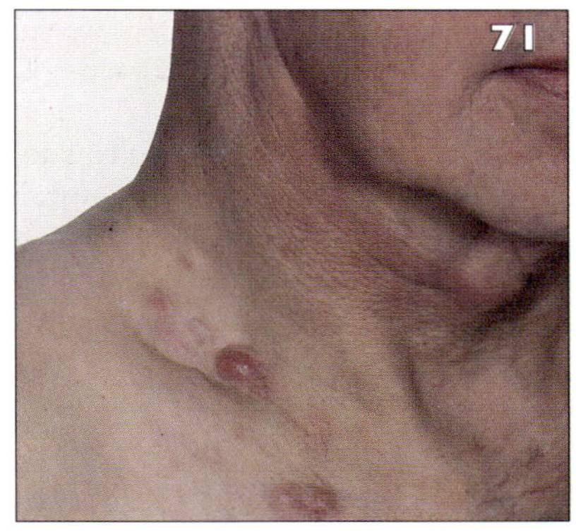

72 An HIV-antibody positive man (CD4+ count of 0.06×10^9/l) has worsening cutaneous Kaposi's sarcoma (KS) which also involves the palate. The chest radiograph showed fine bilateral reticulonodular shadowing. A bronchoscopic alveolar lavage, taken at the same time as the baseline pulmonary function tests, was negative for pathogens, but tracheal and bronchial KS were seen. He received cytotoxic chemotherapy with bleomycin and vincristine in 3-weekly cycles. Eight weeks later he reported increasing exertional dyspnoea and a non-productive cough. There was partial regression of the skin and palatal tumours but the chest radiograph was unchanged. Repeat pulmonary function tests were performed (Table).
i. What is the likely cause of the change in the lung function?
ii. How would you confirm the diagnosis?

Test	Baseline (% predicted)	After 8 weeks (% predicted)
FEV$_1$	98	73
FVC	101	70
TL$_{CO}$*	86	47
K$_{CO}$*	88	63

*Corrected for haemoglobin

73 i. What is shown in 73?
ii. What is it used for?
iii. How useful is it?

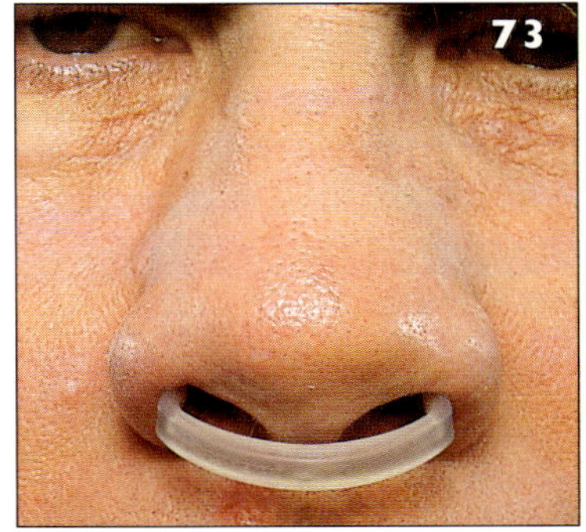

71 i. The lesion shows supraclavicular lymphadenopathy and a further lesion just below the head of the right clavicle. Fine-needle aspiration confirmed small-cell lung cancer.
ii. The treatment of these lesions is with palliative radiotherapy.
iii. Relapse chemotherapy in small-cell lung cancer is generally disappointing. Although chemotherapy as initial treatment may produce response rates of up to 80%, the response rate in relapsed disease is usually less than 20%. There are no clear guidelines as to what chemotherapy to use in relapse. It is reasonable to repeat the initial chemotherapeutic schedule or to use alternative drugs. Most patients who relapse are usually not well enough or unwilling to receive full doses of intravenous 3-weekly cycles of chemotherapy. They may be best treated with single-agent chemotherapy or may be suitable for phase II studies of new cytotoxic agents. In general, the greater the time that has elapsed from the completion of initial treatment to relapse, the greater the chance of the patient responding to further chemotherapy. This is unlikely to be substantial in more than 20% of individuals.

72 i. Possible causes include:
- Progressive Kaposi's sarcoma, but this is unlikely as the skin and palate lesions are regressing on treatment and the chest radiograph is unchanged.
- Bleomycin pulmonary toxicity, but the patient has only received two courses.
- Intercurrent *P. carinii* pneumonia or other infection including pyogenic or mycobacterial causes.

ii. Fibre-optic bronchoscopy. This showed regression of the tracheobronchial Kaposi's sarcoma; cytological examination of the lavage fluid confirmed *P. carinii* pneumonia.

A single reduced TL_{CO} recording cannot distinguish *P. carinii* from other opportunistic infections. A low TL_{CO} can occur in asymptomatic HIV-positive individuals, as well as those with infections and pulmonary KS. A fall in TL_{CO}, from baseline, of >5% when used to predict the presence of *P. carinii* pneumonia has a sensitivity of 75% but a specificity of only 28%. A normal TL_{CO} value is very useful because of the high negative predictive value (98%) which would make *P. carinii* pneumonia unlikely.

73 i. A Nozovent.
ii. Treatment of snoring
iii. It is useful in about 5–10% of snorers, especially in those whose examination shows a substantial opening of the anterior nares on inspiratory nasal flow. Unfortunately it can fall out during the night. It has not been of proven benefit in OSA as most patients with this condition have airway obstruction at sites distal to the anterior nares.

74 i. A 60-year-old man had progressive dyspnoea and bilateral ankle swelling. He was admitted several times over the past year and diagnosed to have 'chronic obstructive airway disease'. Arterial blood gas tensions showed hypercapnic respiratory failure. His chest radiograph was normal. A flow–volume loop was done.
i. What do the spirometry (Table) and flow–volume loop (74) show?
ii. Was the diagnosis correct?
iii. What are the possible causes?
iv. What test would confirm the diagnosis and what does this test involve?

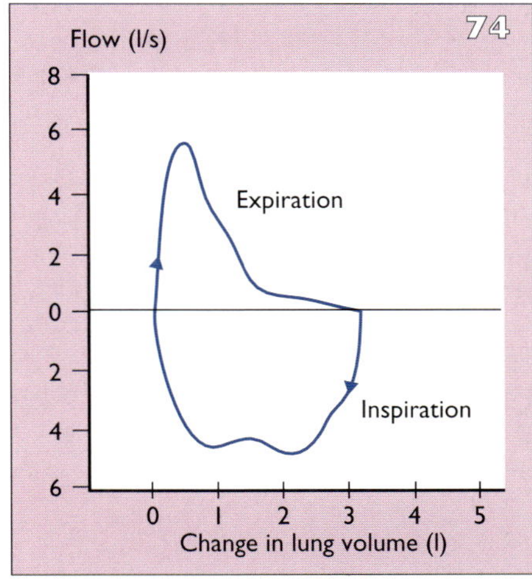

Test	Predicted	Range	Result	% Predicted
PEFR (l/min)	531	451–611	361	68
FEV$_1$ (l)	3.16	2.69–3.63	2.13	67
FVC (l)	4.03	3.43–4.65	3.25	81
FEV$_1$/FVC (%)	71	61–82	65	92

75 This photomicrograph (75) of a Wright–Geimsa-stained cytospin was prepared from BAL fluid obtained from a 54-year-old Middle-Eastern woman with a chronic cough, wheezing and peripheral blood eosinophilia. Her chest radiograph showed mild, diffuse interstitial infiltrates.
i. What cells are present in the BAL?
ii. What diagnoses should be considered?

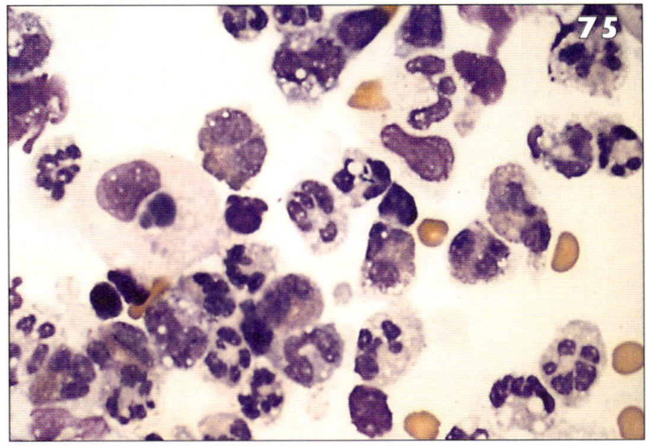

74 i. Mild volume-dependent airway collapse with a FEV_1/FVC of 65%.
ii. No. The mild obstructive airway disease seen on the flow–volume loop by itself is unlikely to explain the respiratory failure.
iii. Central or obstructive sleep apnoea. Respiratory failure usually does not occur in sleep apnoea unless there is concomitant chronic obstructive airway disease, even though this may be very mild.
iv. Polysomnography – this includes continuous monitoring of the electroencephalogram, electro-oculogram and chin electromyogram for sleep staging, continuous monitoring of arterial oxygen saturation with a finger probe using a pulse oximeter, ribcage and abdominal movement to measure apnoeas and hypopnoeas using inductance plethysmography, continuous measurement of nasal airflow using a nasal thermistor, monitoring of body position, monitoring of leg movement and measurement of snoring using a microphone. There is no respiratory effort during the period of absent airflow at the nose and mouth in central sleep apnoea in contrast to obstructive sleep apnoea.

75 i. The BAL shows numerous eosinophils (in addition to neutrophils and alveolar macrophages) suggesting an allergic process such as asthma, allergic bronchopulmonary aspergillosis or chronic eosinophilic pneumonia.
ii. The patient's tropical origin makes parasitic infection an important consideration. Occult filariasis is also called pulmonary infiltrates with eosinophilia (i.e. the PIE syndrome) or tropical pulmonary eosinophilia. It manifests as intermittent coughing, wheezing, and vague systemic symptoms. Lymphadenopathy may be seen but massive lymphoedema is absent. Radiographic features are variable and include interstitial, miliary or focal consolidative patterns. Eosinophilia is routinely present and serum IgE levels are markedly increased. Occult filariasis is thought to represent an allergic reaction to the circulating microfilaria of the mosquito-borne nematodes, *Wuchereria bancrofti* and *Brugai malayi*. A sustained hypersensitivity reaction leads to interstitial lung injury, eosinophilic and granulomatous infiltration, and fibrosis. The diagnosis of occult filariasis is supported by findings of eosinophilia, elevated IgE levels and positive serology in a patient with a compatible clinical presentation. Microfilariae may be seen in the lung or lymph nodes but, if the diagnosis is suspected, a therapeutic trial of diethylcarbamazine is preferable to biopsy.

76 Over the preceding 6 months this patient has complained of chronic cough which temporarily improved somewhat on antibiotics. He now complains of fever, breathlessness and a productive cough with purulent sputum for 2 weeks. The CD4+ lymphocyte count is 0.02×10^9/l.
i. What are the abnormalities in the two radiographs **76a** and **76b**?
ii. Are these two conditions related and if so what is the likely aetiology?
iii. Describe an appropriate management plan for the acute condition.
iv. How commonly is the condition in radiograph (**76b**) seen in HIV-positive patients and what are the causes?

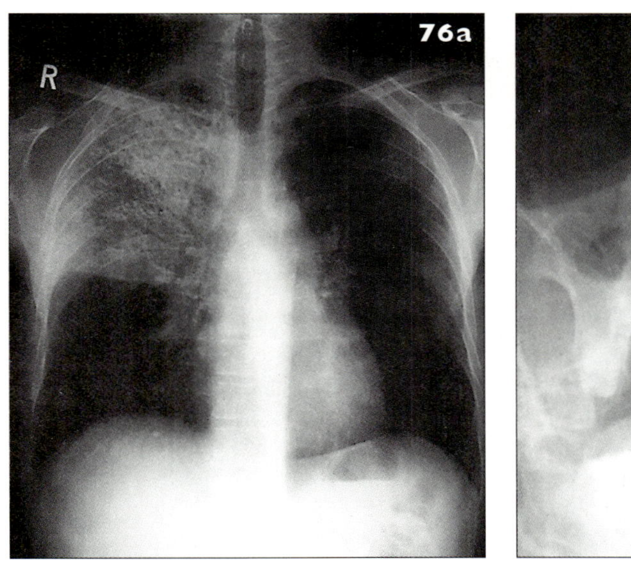

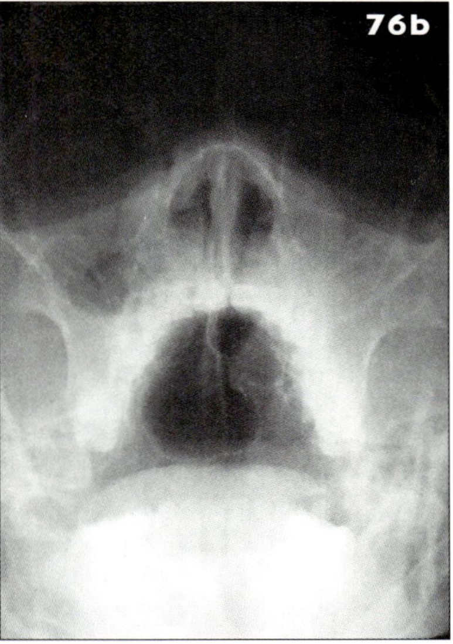

77 What are some broad predictors to identify patients who may be successfully weaned from a ventilator.

76 i. The chest film shows lobar shadowing consistent with acute infection. The sinus views in (**76b**) show mucosal thickening and sinus opacification indicative of chronic sinusitis.

ii. The history of chronic cough in this setting is probably due to a post-nasal drip related to chronic sinusitis and rhinitis. The more acute illness is suggestive of a bacterial chest infection, although other aetiologies such as *P. carinii* should still be considered. Chronic inflammation of the frontal, maxillary and ethmoid sinuses is increasingly associated with acute or sub-acute pneumonia due to *P. aeruginosa*.

iii. The aetiology of the chest infection should be confirmed by sputum culture or bronchoalveolar lavage if necessary, and treated with an anti-pseudomonal antibiotic such as ceftazadime or ciprofloxacin for 2 weeks. There is a high (35%) rate of relapse in these very immunocompromised patients.

iv. Chronic sinusitis is being increasingly recognized as an HIV-associated condition with approximately 5% of patients with a CD4 count under $0.02 \times 10^9/l$ complaining of sinusitis and 15% of AIDS patients having sinus thickening on MRI scanning. The sinusitis is usually related to chronic rhinitis, which should be treated with nasal decongestants and topical steroids. Secondary infection of the sinuses can be acute and related to *H. influenzae* or *Str. pneumoniae*, or indolent and due to pseudomonas. There are recent reports of sinus infection with *Microsporidia* sp.

77 Patients whose lungs were normal before ventilation can be weaned rapidly; however, the process may be protracted in patients with pre-existing lung disease. Patients should require an FiO_2 of no more than 0.4 while having an arterial PaO_2 of >10 kPa (65 mmHg), and have no residual effects of sedatives or muscle relaxants. The underlying condition for which they were initially ventilated should be improving and there should be no other major organ failure. Patients should be able to generate a maximum inspiratory pressure of at least –20 cmH_2O.

78 Shown are the chest radiograph (78a) and chest CT (78b) of a 34-year-old man with symptoms of a non-productive cough and occasional, scant haemoptysis. He had received a full course of treatment for pulmonary tuberculosis 2 years earlier.
i. What are the radiographic findings?
ii. What is the most likely diagnosis?
iii. What management approach is indicated?

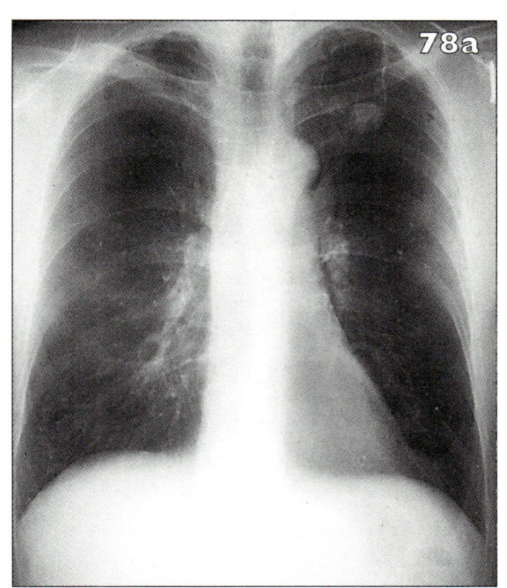

79 An elderly patient with COPD is planning a trip involving air travel. He asks if he will need oxygen during the flight.
i. What is the effective cabin altitude inside most pressurized commercial aircraft when cruising at peak altitude?
ii. If, at sea level breathing air this patient's arterial blood gas showed a pH of 7.39, a pCO_2 of 6.5 kPa (41 mmHg), and pO_2 of 8.5 kPa (62 mmHg), would you prescribe supplemental O_2 for his flight?

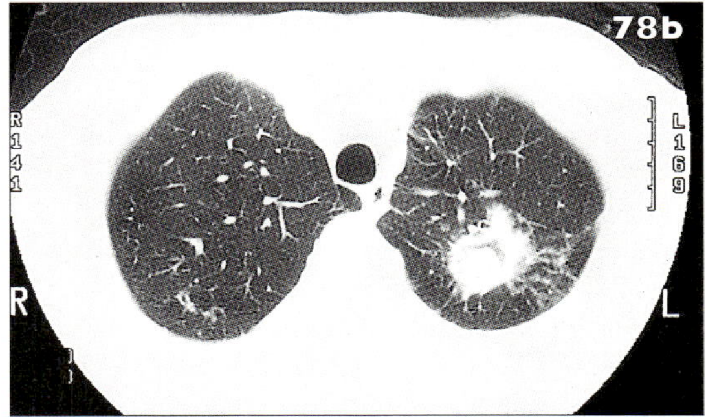

78 i. 78a and **78b** show an irregular, thin-walled cavity containing a nodular density in the dependent position. There are some linear streaks extending toward the hilum but no surrounding infiltrates.

ii. This is most likely an aspergilloma (also called a mycetoma or a fungus ball) growing in a pre-existing lung cavity. Classically the mass is described as having an 'air-halo'.

iii. Aspergilloma are common, and a complication of tuberculous cavities and patients with chronic sarcoid cavities. Most are asymptomatic and the problem may be discovered as an incidental radiographic finding. Serum precipitins against *Aspergillus* species are usually elevated. Haemoptysis can be the presenting manifestation and, on occasion, may be life-threatening. Although most aspergillomas are saprophytic, rather than invasive infections, immunosuppressed patients may develop a locally invasive form of the disease extending into the lung tissue adjacent to an aspergilloma, a form of chronic necrotizing aspergillosis. Most aspergilloma require no treatment. Excision is very difficult due to adhesions around the affected lobe and because of the underlying chronic lung disease. Angiographic embolization is another option for haemoptysis, but is also difficult as the bronchial artery supplying the cavity is not hypertrophied – as in cystic fibrosis. Selected patients may benefit from intracavitary amphotericin B or oral itraconazole. Systemic antifungal treatment with amphotericin B should be instituted promptly in patients with chronic necrotizing aspergillosis.

79 i. Most commercial aircraft cruise at between 22 000 ft (6706 m) and 44 000 ft (13 411 m) above sea level. Pressurization is added to the cabin to yield an effective cabin altitude of 5000 ft (1529 m) to 8000 ft (2438 m) at most cruising altitudes. The P_IO_2 is approximately 21 kPa (150 mmHg) at sea level and falls to 17 kPa (118 mmHg) at 8000 ft (2438 m). At 8000–10 000 ft, the corresponding arterial partial pressure of oxygen (PaO_2) is 6.5–7.9 kPa (50–60 mmHg) in most healthy individuals at rest.

ii. Yes. Supplemental O_2 should be prescribed because his pre-flight, sea level, room air PaO_2 is <10 kPa (70 mmHg). Ideally it is difficult to arrange for flows of 4 l/min of oxygen on intercontinental flights.

Altitude simulation tests may be performed to assist in O_2 prescription. Patients inhale FiO_2 of 0.18 or 0.16 either at rest or with light exercise, to determine if any oxygen desaturation can be corrected by 2 or 4 l/min of oxygen.

80 This 30-year-old man complains of mild exertional dyspnoea.
i. Of what condition is the chest radiograph on inspiration (**80a**) and expiration (**80b**) suggestive, and what is the possible aetiology?
ii. From what else should the condition be distinguished?

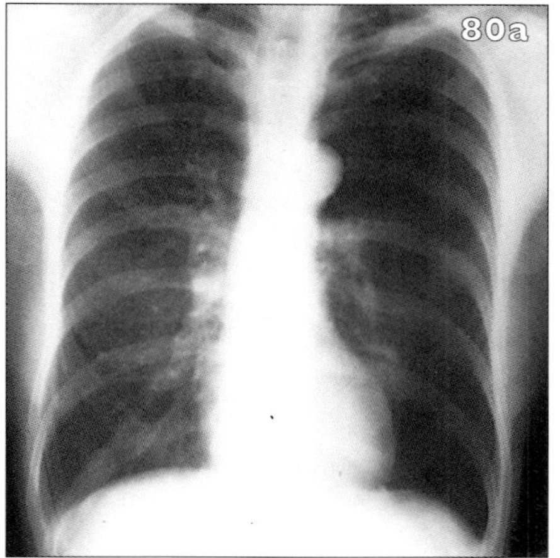 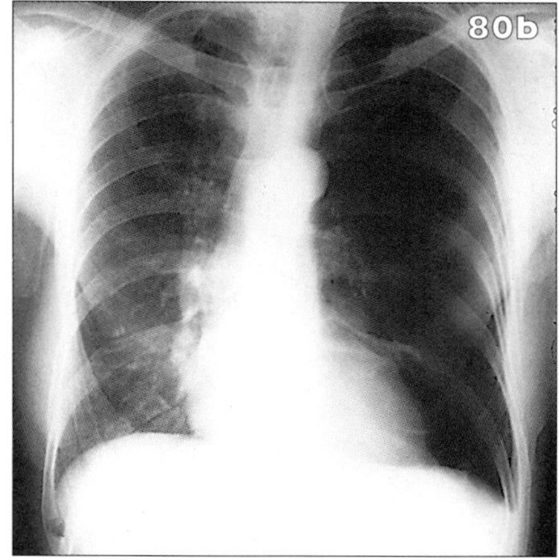

81 A patient with known carcinoma of the bronchus presents with a 2-day history of progressive mid-lumbar back pain and numbness on the anterior surface of the left thigh. Shown (**81a**) is his lateral lumbar spine radiograph.
i. What is the likely cause of the symptoms?
ii. How would you investigate them?
iii. How would you treat the patient?

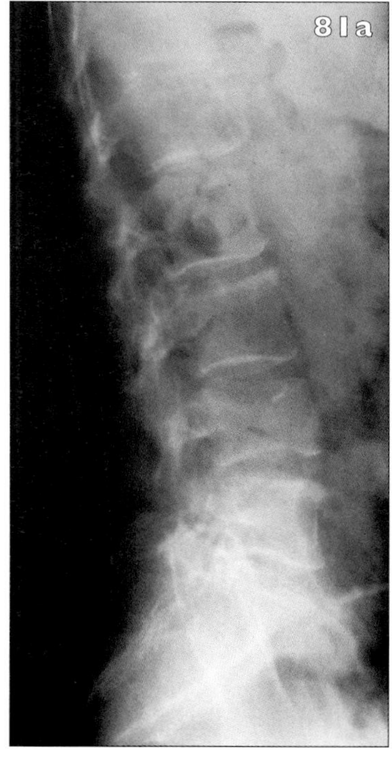

80 i. The radiographic finding of a unilateral radiolucent lung was described by Macleod and is also known as Swyer–James syndrome. The syndrome is ascribed to neonatal or early childhood bronchiolitis obliterans. The lung is usually otherwise normal and well-preserved, but with small pulmonary vessels. Large air spaces can develop, with poor ventilation of the affected lung, which may remain fully inflated on an expiratory film (80b). The prognosis is good.

ii. Other causes of a radiolucent appearance to a lung include congenital absence of the chest wall muscles or mastectomy, obstruction to a pulmonary artery by embolus or tumour, compression of the pulmonary artery by tumour or nodes and congenital abnormalities. Partial obstruction of a main bronchus by a tumour or a foreign body can occasionally produce unilateral hyperlucensy.

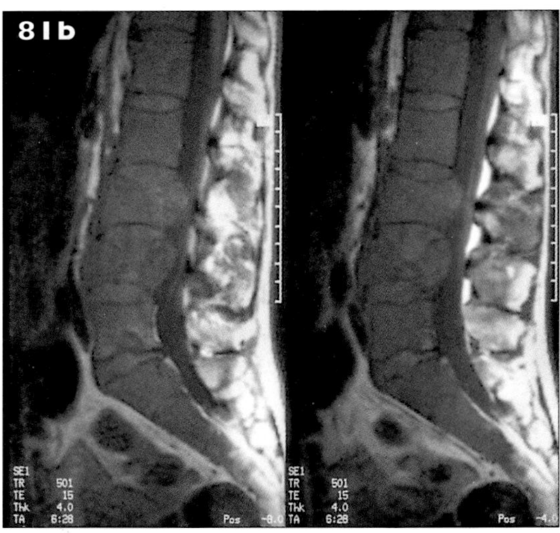

81 i. The back pain is most likely to be due to metastatic disease. The vertebral column is one of the most common sites of metastatic spread.

ii. The numbness of the thigh may indicate a root lesion (lower motor neurone) compatible with early corda equina compression. Enquiries as to bladder and other sphincter function is essential. The patient needs plain radiographs of the lower thoracic and lumbar spine. Even if normal, further investigation is needed. If the radiographic changes are suggestive of metastatic disease, i.e. loss of height of a vertebral body or loss of a pedicle, one should proceed to examination of the spinal column, ideally by MRI scan to see the spinal cord, the bony structures and any soft tissue mass due to tumour (81b).

If the plain spinal radiographs are normal, then a bone scan should be performed and, if abnormal in the area under suspicion, one should then proceed to MRI scan. If the MRI is not immediately available, then myelography is an excellent investigation to perform.

iii. Suspected paraparesis needs urgent treatment. Paraplegia, once established, rarely improves. Primary treatment is radiotherapy together with steroid cover. There is no advantage from surgical decompression.

In patients with small-cell lung cancer, if the cord lesion is the presenting symptom, then chemotherapy can be added following radiotherapy if the clinical response appears adequate.

82 Shown (**82a**) is the chest radiograph of a 29-year-old, non-smoking woman with severe steroid-dependent asthma. She had symptoms of dyspnoea, wheezing, and a cough which was productive of thick mucous and small plugs. A left upper lobe pneumonia occurred 3 months earlier during an exacerbation of asthma and cleared with a course of antibiotics and an increase in her steroid dose.

i. Describe the radiographic findings.

ii. Discuss the most likely explanation for this clinical presentation.

iii. Outline an appropriate diagnostic and therapeutic approach.

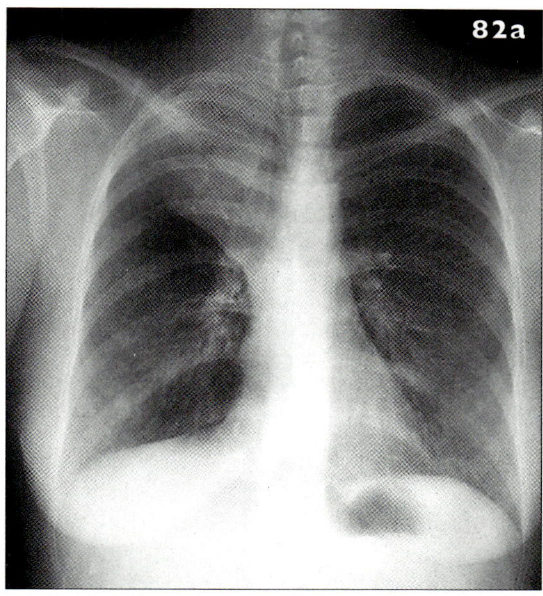

83 A patient is receiving nebulized 3% saline.

i. What type of nebulizer is being used (**83**)?

ii. What are the indications for the use of 3% saline?

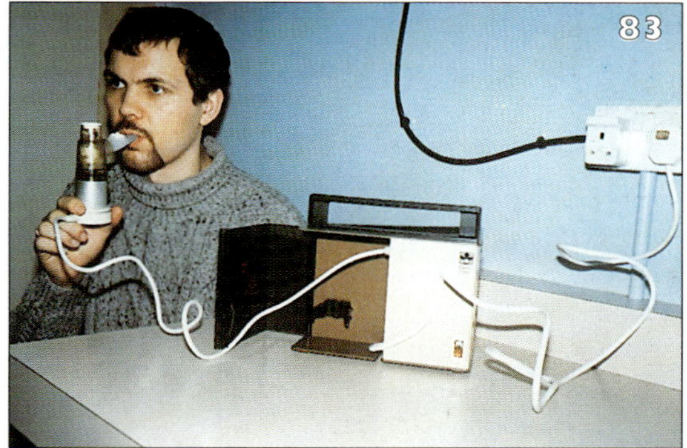

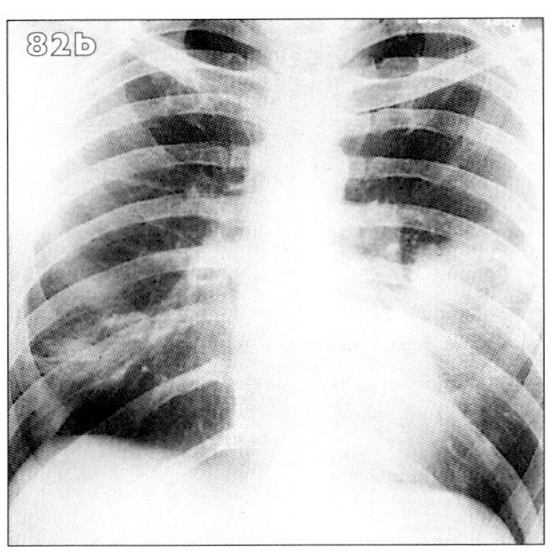

82 i. The chest radiograph (**82a**) shows some hyperinflation of the left lung with right upper lobe consolidation and collapse. There is some peribronchial cuffing.

ii. The radiographic changes, together with the clinical history, should suggest the diagnosis of allergic bronchopulmonary aspergillosis (ABPA). ABPA is characterized by reversible airflow obstruction, recurrent lung infiltrates and fever, eosinophilia, mucous plugs and central bronchiectasis. Often, eosinophils and mould hyphae are present in the sputum, and moulds may be cultured from the sputum. Serum IgE levels are usually markedly elevated and aspergillus-specific hypersensitivity can be confirmed by skin reactivity or by specific anti-aspergillus IgE titres. Bronchiectasis occurs at a relatively late stage of the disease. Subsequent exacerbations can cause extensive damage (**82b**).

iii. The evaluation of patients with asthma and lobar collapse and/or pulmonary infiltrates should include a differential blood count and serum IgE level. Sputum should be examined for eosinophils and for hyphae, and cultured for fungi. Specific anti-aspergillus IgE titres and skin testing can be confirmatory. Bronchiectasis can be identified with greater sensitivity by high-resolution CT scanning than by plain radiographs. The treatment of ABPA typically requires systemic corticosteroids. Once the pulmonary infiltrate has cleared the patient's medication should be determined only by the severity of the asthma and oral steroids stopped if possible.

83 i. This is an ultrasonic nebulizer. It uses high-frequency sound waves from a piezoelectric crystal impacting on the surface of the liquid in the reservoir to generate a fountain of droplets. A baffle above this fountain collects the larger droplets, leaving a mist of smaller droplets to be inhaled by the patient. Usually no driving gas is used. The solution is warmed by the effect of the sound waves. The output of drug from this nebulizer is usually greater than for jet nebulizers so that the same quantity of drug can be delivered more quickly. The size of particle generated is larger with this type of nebulizer (5–10 μm), and the fraction of particles likely to be exhaled (up to 2 μm) is less than with jet nebulizers.

ii. As 3% saline is hypertonic it draws fluid into alveoli and peripheral airways, as well as facilitating expectoration by an irritant effect on major bronchi. It is therefore useful for sputum induction, usually for diagnostic purposes, for example in detecting *P. carinii*, although it is not as sensitive as bronchoscopy for this purpose. Problems in some patients include nausea, bronchospasm, and oxygen desaturation.

84 A 38-year-old man is being evaluated for fitness as a fire-fighter. His heart rate and ventilatory responses to exercise expressed as increasing oxygen uptake are shown in **84a** and **84b**.
i. Does he have a normal heart rate response to exercise?
ii. What is his maximal oxygen uptake? Is it normal?
iii. Why does the ventilatory response have an inflection towards the end of the test?

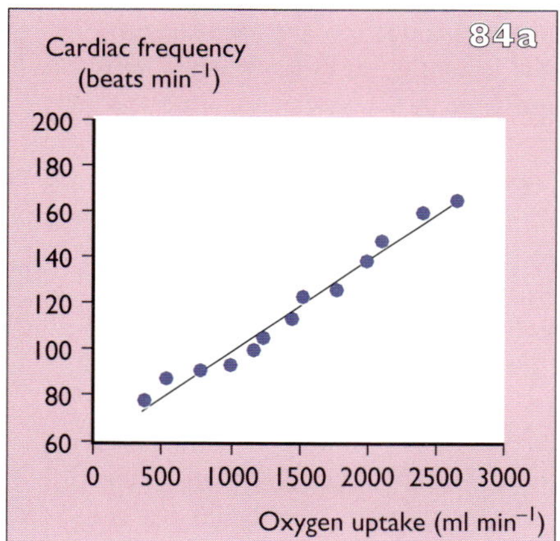

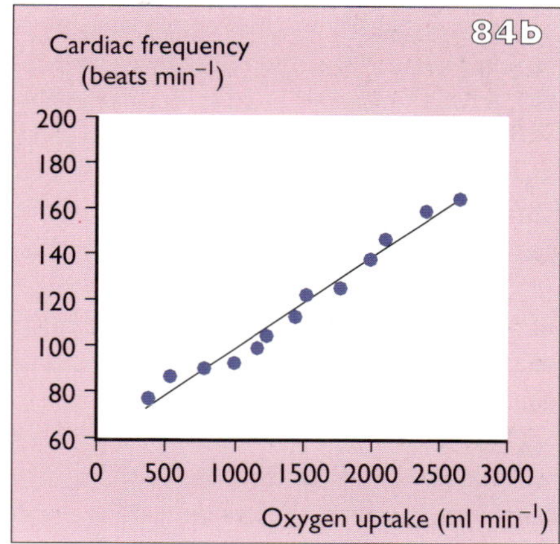

85 This radiograph (**85a**) of a 25-year-old man was taken on admission to hospital via the accident and emergency department and a second film (**85b**) was taken 3 weeks later in the intensive care unit. From the changes seen on the two chest radiographs, what is the most likely diagnosis?

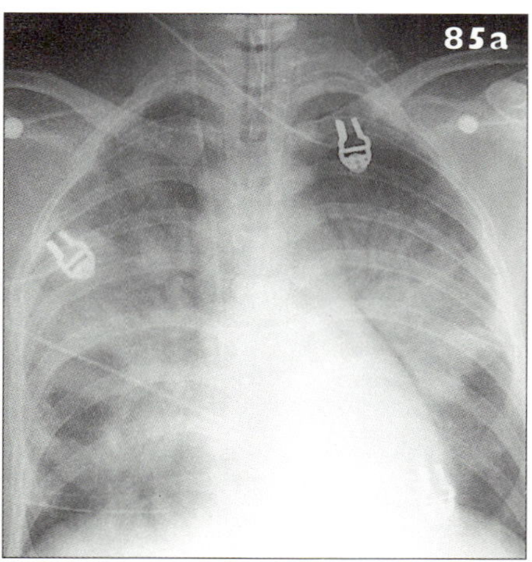

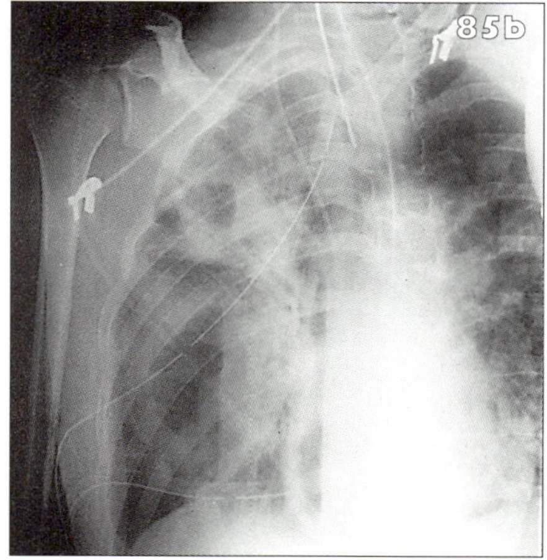

84 i. The heart rate response to exercise is linear and exercise would normally continue with a steady increase in heart rate as the oxygen uptake demand increases. The patient stopped exercise with a heart rate of 170 beats/min, which is 85% of the maximum predicted for a man of this age. Many exercise tests are stopped in patients when the heart rate reaches 85% of the predicted normal. The maximum predicted heart rate is 210 minus 6 beats per 10 years of age from the age of 20.
ii. The maximal oxygen uptake is 2.5 l/min. The maximal oxygen uptake in normal subjects varies enormously with their age, weight and general aerobic capacity, i.e. fitness. The oxygen uptake shown (**84b**), i.e. at 85% of maximum predicted heart rate, is within the normal range and represents a good response by the patient.
iii. Ventilation also increases linearly with oxygen uptake and CO_2 output. However, as exercise approaches maximal, anaerobic metabolism becomes an important factor and the resultant metabolic acidosis causes an additional ventilatory stimulus. It is, therefore, common to see an inflection in the ventilatory response to exercise at the 'anaerobic threshold'. This is shown in this fire-fighter's response to occur during the last minute of exercise and is a normal feature.

85 Radiograph **85a** shows multiple rib fractures on the right side with a chest drain *in situ*, bilateral alveolar infiltrates and a pneumo-mediastinum as indicated by the rim of gas outlining the left heart border.

The unifying diagnosis in this case is trauma and the patient was a victim of a road traffic accident 36 hours earlier. The lung infiltrates could be due to aspiration but more probably represent ARDS resulting from increased permeability of the pulmonary alveolar capillary membrane, as a result of blunt trauma. Pulmonary contusion is another possibility. Other causes of pneumo-mediastinum include penetrating chest injuries, damage to the upper airway during instrumentation and tracheostomy formation, oesophageal rupture or perforation and, rarely, gastrointestinal tract perforation below the diaphragm with air tracking up to the mediastinum via the retroperitoneal tissues. However, the most common cause is alveolar rupture due to high alveolar pressures. Air may track up the mediastinum to produce surgical emphysema of the face, neck, supraclavicular areas and upper chest. This particularly applies during intermittent positive-pressure ventilation in severe asthma and in ARDS where poor compliance of the lungs results in increased alveolar pressures. It is also reported after vomiting, straining at stool, parturition and performing a Valsalva manoeuvre. It is frequently symptomless but may cause central chest pain and auscultation may reveal a clicking sound during systole (Hamman's sign). The mediastinal air can often be seen more impressively on a lateral chest radiograph.

86 i. Of what is this appearance (86) a part? In which cell type of lung cancer does this occur and what is the treatment of choice?
ii. What other hormone-secreting effects are seen commonly in lung cancer?

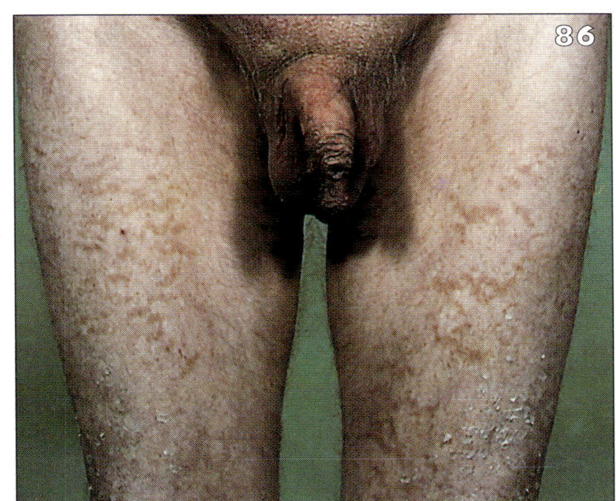

87 The worker shown (87) is filing a tungsten carbide saw.
i. What respiratory diseases are associated with 'hard-metal' exposure?
ii. What is the causative agent?
iii. What is the usual clinical course of this disease?
iv. What other metals are associated with interstitial fibrosis?

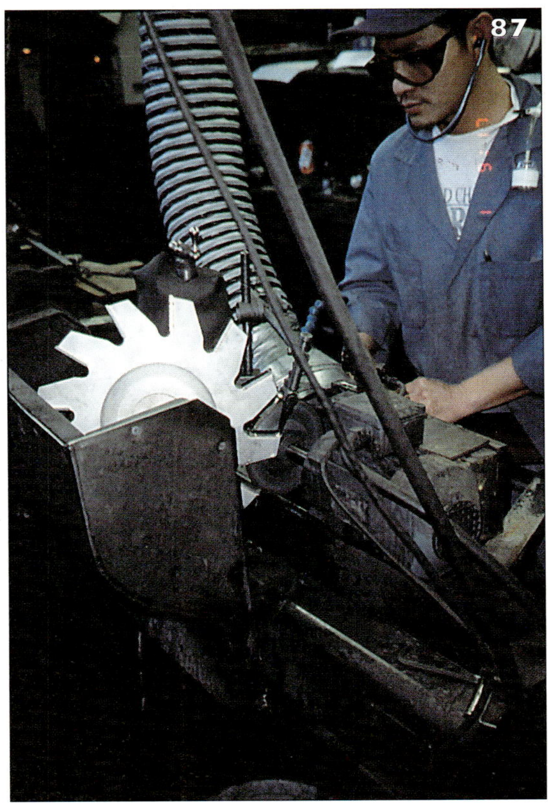

86 i. The illustration (86) is of pigmented striae, in a man with small-cell lung cancer who has ectopic ACTH secretion. The plasma ACTH levels are elevated in up to 30% of patients presenting with small-cell lung cancer, but the natural history of the disease is too short to allow florid Cushing's syndrome to develop. Occasionally, pigmentation – as shown here – is seen together with thirst, proximal myopathy, hypokalaemic alkalosis, and elevated plasma cortisol. The treatment is of the underlying tumour with cytotoxic chemotherapy.

ii. The most common syndrome is inappropriate anti-diuretic hormone secretion (SIADH) and is exclusive to small-cell lung cancer. The patient initially retains water but eventually becomes clinically dehydrated. The serum urea, sodium and osmolarity are low with a concentrated urine with a osmolarity at least 2.5-fold that of the serum. It occurs as a clinical problem in 10–15% of new cases of SCLC. A water loading excretion test is abnormal in 60% of patients. Hypercalcaemia also occurs from the secretion of a parathormone-like peptide from primary squamous cell tumour.

87 i. Hard-metal lung disease classically refers to interstitial lung disease occurring in individuals manufacturing or working with cemented tungsten carbide tools. In addition, these workers may also develop occupational asthma, hypersensitivity pneumonitis, giant cell interstitial pneumonitis and bronchiolitis obliterans. There may be a continuum of disease with components of several processes present simultaneously in an affected individual.

ii. Cobalt, a binding agent used in the manufacturing process, rather than tungsten carbide is the causal agent. Tungsten carbide is relatively non-toxic in animals and characteristic hard-metal lung disease occurs in workers exposed to cobalt alone. The presence of tungsten but occasional absence of cobalt in lung biopsies of hard metal workers reflects the high solubility of cobalt and rapid transit out of the lung.

iii. A minority of exposed workers develop disease. Cough, wheezing and dyspnoea are typical early symptoms though fever, chills and malaise suggestive of extrinsic allergic alveolitis may be present. Initially, patients improve when removed from the workplace but continued exposure leads to chronic, progressive impairment. Reduced lung volumes and diffusion capacity are typical pulmonary function abnormalities of patients with chronic disease. The latency between first exposure and onset of disease may range from 6 months to 4 years.

iv. Metals are associated with numerous pulmonary airway and parenchymal disorders. Interstitial fibrosis may occur following exposure to aluminium, barium, beryllium, cadmium, copper, gold, mercury, nickel, thallium, titanium, zinc, and the rare earth metals (cerium, yttrium, terbium).

88 Shown (88) is the result of a surgical procedure on the oropharynx.
i. Which procedure was performed and what does it treat?
ii. What are the non-surgical methods available to treat this problem?

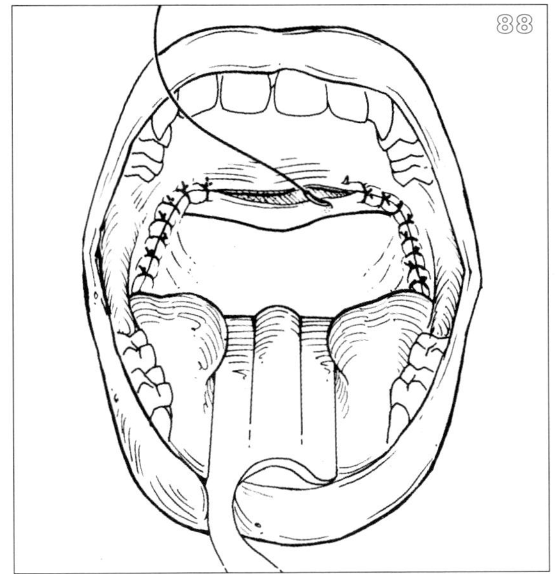

89 These radiographs (89a, 89b) are of a 32-year-old man with cough, sputum, recurrent chest infections, sinusitis and partial deafness.
i. What are the abnormalities shown?
ii. What is the condition and what is the major defect?
iii. Describe the management.
iv. What is the mode of inheritance? Name other similar conditions.

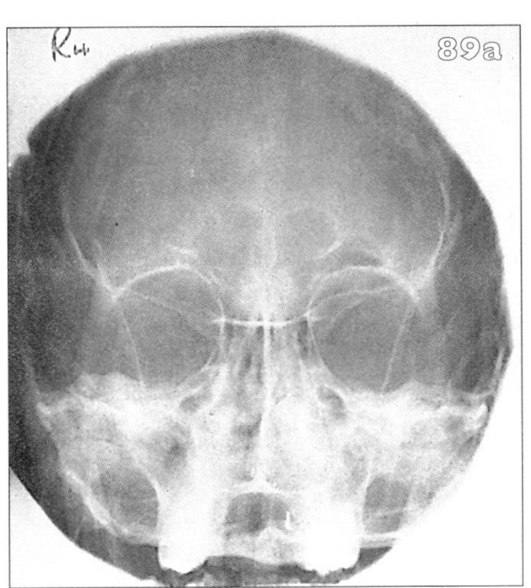

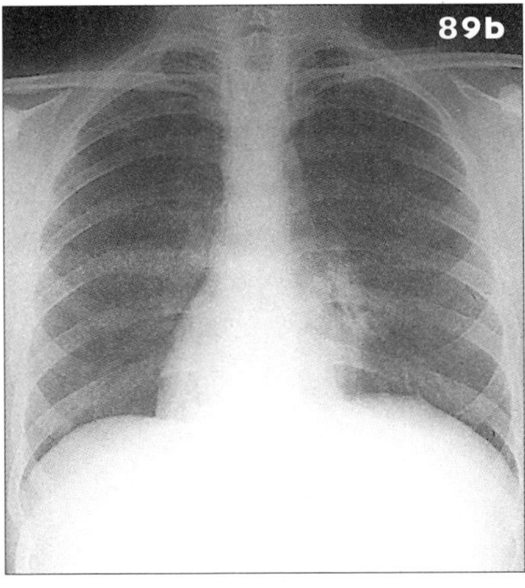

88 i. Uvulopalatopharyngoplasty (UPPP) increases the size of the oropharyngeal lumen by removing redundant soft tissue. It involves removing a small portion of the soft palate and uvula and any tonsillar tissue which is present. Its most appropriate role is in the treatment of snoring that occurs in the *absence* of OSA. UPPP has also been used to treat OSA, but with low efficacy. If patients are appropriately selected (i.e. those with obstruction at the pharyngeal level due to a long soft palate, to redundant pharyngeal wall and/or to excess tonsillar tissue), a majority will experience at least a 50% reduction in respiratory events. In most instances the operation does not cure moderate or severe OSA because obstruction is present at other levels in addition to the pharynx. The danger in performing UPPP for snoring in unscreened patients is that coexisting OSA may go untreated.

ii. Non-surgical methods which can be effective in treating snoring include: weight loss, avoidance of sedatives (including alcohol) before sleep, avoiding the supine position during sleep (a tennis ball sewn on the back of nightware may be helpful), and the use of tongue-retaining and dental devices.

89 i. The facial radiograph (**89a**) shows no air in the frontal sinuses and gross mucosal thickening of the maxillary sinuses, especially the left. The chest radiograph (**89b**) shows dextrocardia.

ii. The patient has Kartagener's syndrome (also known as the ciliary dyskinesia syndrome) with poorly developed or absent frontal sinuses, chronic sinusitis, situs invertus (in 50% of cases), eventual bronchiectasis and immotile cilia – both in the respiratory tract and sperm immotility. The structural defect in the cilia include absence of dynein arms, radial spokes or microtubules. Because of abnormal ciliary movement, mucus collects in the bronchi, sinuses and Eustachian tubes causing cough, infected sputum, ultimately bronchiectasis, sinusitis and deafness. Infertility is common in males.

iii. The treatment is that of chronic bronchial sepsis with broad-spectrum antibiotics when necessary, postural drainage of bronchiectatic areas; grommets and antrostomies for the ear and nasal problems. The prognosis is good.

iv. Primary ciliac dyskinesia is autosomally recessive with incomplete penetrance, and occurs with a frequency of 1 in 15 000 to 1 in 30 000. Young described a syndrome in males of obstructive azoospermia, sinusitis and bronchiectasis. Secondary ciliary dyskinesia occurs when normal cilia beat more slowly; this can occur in severe asthma, viral infections, bacterial infections and with heavy tobacco consumption.

90 Shown is a representative high-power photomicrograph (90) of a Wright–Geimsa-stained cytospin prepared from BAL fluid from a patient with interstitial lung disease.
i. What cell types are present?
ii. Discuss the interaction of these cells in lung inflammation.

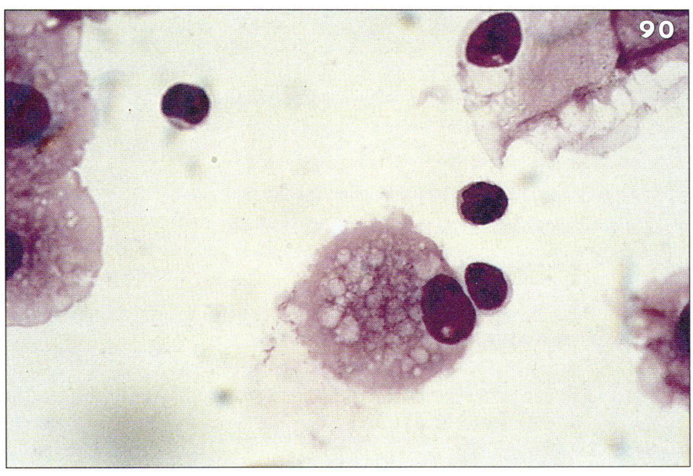

91 i. What is the diagnosis of the condition shown in **91** and what are the symptoms?
ii. What are the predisposing factors?
iii. What is the relationship between asthma and sinus disease?

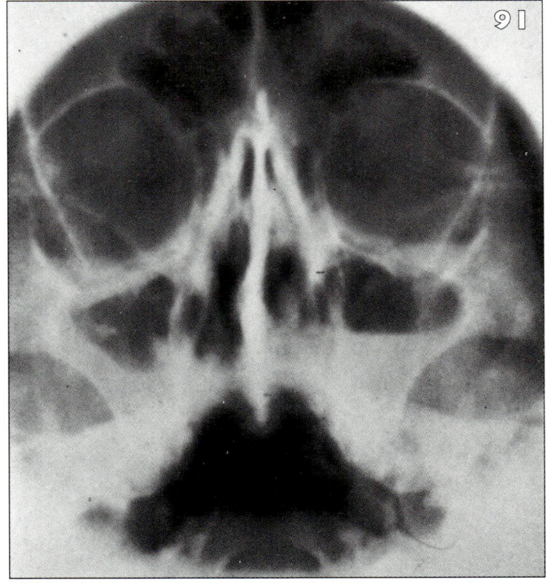

90 i. This BAL specimen contains predominantly alveolar macrophages and lymphocytes (the smaller cells).

ii. Lymphocytes are key cells in the cognate arm of the immune system, reacting to specific antigenic determinants rather than to generalized, non-specific stimuli. Most lymphocytes in the lung are T-cells which participate in the delayed type hypersensitivity and cytotoxic responses of cell-mediated immunity. The remainder are B-cells, responsible for antibody production in the humoral response, and other miscellaneous subsets. T-cells are central to host defence against viral and other intracellular pathogens and to the immune surveillance for malignancy. They augment macrophage antimicrobial and tumoricidal effects and directly lyse host cells bearing microbial or antigens. T-lymphocytes recognizing a persistent environmental antigen or self antigen can contribute to the lung injury characteristic of a myriad of immunologically mediated lung diseases including asthma and virtually all of the interstitial lung diseases. T-cell subpopulations in BAL fluid may be characterized as to their cell-surface marker phenotype. Cells expressing CD4 are called T-helper lymphocytes and cells expressing CD8 are called T-suppresser lymphocytes. Identification of the relative proportions of CD4- and CD8-positive cells in a lymphocytic alveolitis has been used to help distinguish among different types of interstitial lung disease. Sarcoidosis is typically associated with a high CD4/CD8 ratio whereas hypersensitivity pneumonitis usually results in a low ratio. There may be considerable overlap in these criteria, however, which may complicate using this ratio when evaluating an individual patient.

91 i. Paranasal sinusitis. There is bilateral mucosal thickening and air-fluid levels in the maxillary sinuses, worse on the left. Symptoms include headache, pain and tenderness over the affected sinuses, periorbital swelling in children, nasal congestion and obstruction, purulent nasal secretions, postnasal drainage, cough, sore throat and purulent sputum. CT scan of the paranasal sinuses is very sensitive and specific means of showing sinus disease.

ii. Predisposing factors include acute viral, bacterial, mycoplasma or other respiratory tract infections, foreign bodies, nasogastric or nasotracheal tubes, nasal packing, exposures to respiratory tract irritants, barotrauma associated with flying, swimming and diving. More long-standing risk factors include allergic rhinitis, nasal polyposis, immunoglobulin deficiencies, AIDS, anatomical disorders, cystic fibrosis or the ciliary dyskinesia syndrome.

iii. Sinusitis is a frequent finding in patients with asthma and can lead to a worsening of asthma. Sinusitis with nasal mucosal congestion and oedema results in decreased humidification and temperature rectification of inhaled air. Sinusitis is associated with postnasal drainage which can carry bacteria and/or inflammatory material to the lower respiratory tract. Asthma and sinusitis are also linked through a common allergic response pathway or a aspirin sensitivity.

92 These are the chest radiograph
(**92a**) and bronchoscopic (**92b**)
appearance of a 24-year-old girl in
whom systemic lupus erythematosus
had been diagnosed 6 months earlier.
Her initial joint symptoms and rash
had been successfully controlled on
steroids but 4 weeks before admission
to ICU she developed symptoms
suggestive of cerebral involvement
and the steroid dose was increased.
She was admitted with respiratory
distress, circulatory collapse and
disseminated intravascular coagulation (DIC). Gram-negative sepsis was
confirmed and she improved with
antibiotic and standard supportive
therapy. Pulsed cyclophosphamide
was subsequently started for lupus
cerebritis diagnosed at MRI scanning.
Several weeks later she suffered a
massive haemoptysis and the chest
radiograph and bronchoscopy were
performed at this time. Similar lesions
to those pictured were present
throughout the bronchial tree.

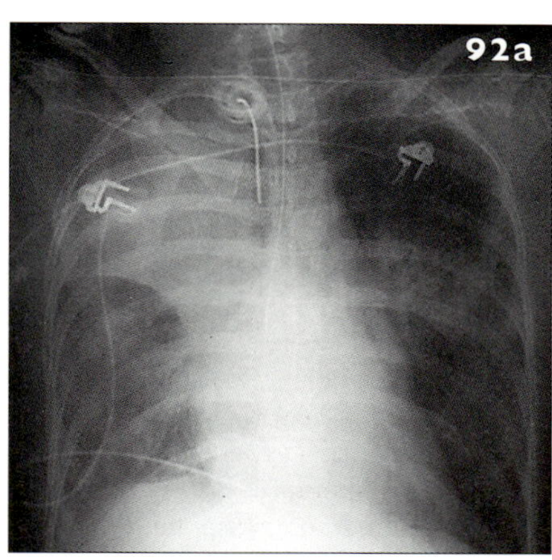

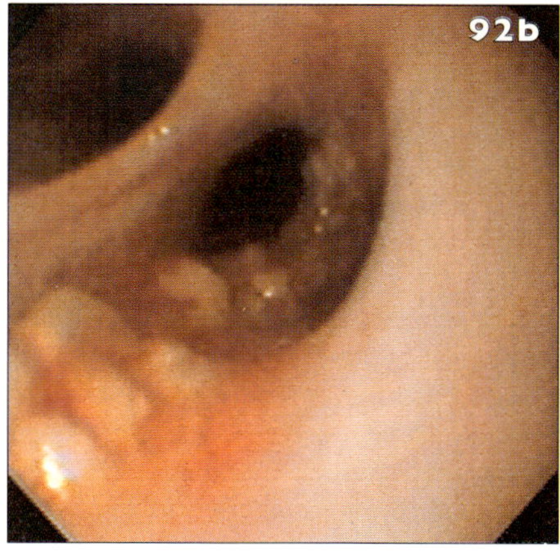

i. Describe the bronchoscopic
appearances.
ii. Which organism is likely to be responsible for the respiratory problems?

93 This 45-year-old white
woman (**93**) presented with
bilateral hilar
lymphadenopathy on chest
radiograph and this painful
rash.

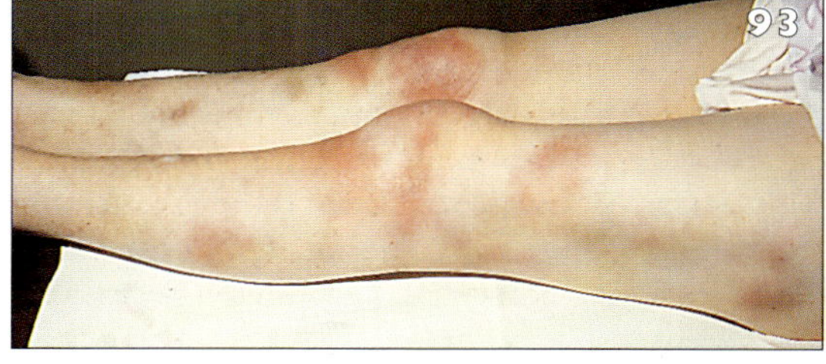

i. What is this syndrome
called?
ii. What is her prognosis?
iii. What other cutaneous manifestations may occur in this disease?

92 i. The chest radiograph shows (**92a**) a densely consolidated right upper lobe with infiltrates in the middle and lower lobes. The bronchoscopy (**92b**) shows mucosal infiltration with white, nodular lesions, suggestive of a fungal infection.

ii. Histology of the bronchial biopsies showed extensive infiltration with fungal hyphae but minimal inflammatory infiltrate. *A. fumigatus* was subsequently isolated. The diagnosis is invasive aspergillosis, an important complication in immunocompromised patients. It usually presents as a necrotizing cavitating pneumonia unresponsive to standard antibiotics. The pulmonary features in this case are rare but a wide variety of presentations have been described. Diagnosis may be difficult with both sputum culture and serology frequently being negative. Biopsy specimens are usually required to make the diagnosis. Extrapulmonary dissemination to the liver, kidney, gastrointestinal tract and brain occurs in about 25% of cases.

Treatment was with intravenous liposomal and nebulized amphoteracin followed by oral itraconazole. The patient recovered, and a follow-up chest radiograph at 3 months was normal.

Aspergillus species can affect the lungs in several ways:

- Allergic bronchopulmonary aspergillosis in asthma (see **82**).
- Aspergilloma – i.e. a fungus ball infects pre-existing cavities (see **78**).
- Invasive aspergillosis, as in this case.
- Aspergillosis pneumonia.
- Tracheal infection.

The last three develop in immunocompromised hosts.

93 i. Lofgren's syndrome, after a Swedish physician who described this in 1946. It consists of bilateral hilar lymphadenopathy and the rash of erythema nodosum. Lymphoma and granulomatous infections should be considered. An elevated serum ACE may reduce the need for a biopsy confirmation in the absence of atypical features. The syndrome usually occurs in young women who often present with fever, malaise, arthralgias and painful lesions on their legs (probably due to circulating immune complexes). The condition occasionally relapses and is uncommon in men.

ii. This woman is in the best prognostic group in whites with a 90% chance of spontaneous remission or her sarcoidosis within 2 years without corticosteroids. The erythema nodosum should fade within weeks.

iii. Cutaneous involvement with sarcoidosis may occur on the anterior surface of the legs with erythema nodosum. The most common other skin manifestations are papulonodular lesions. Nodules are smooth reddish-brown, often solitary or in small groups whereas papules are often numerous and often on the face or neck. Lupus pernio occurs mainly in older women and more commonly in blacks and is associated with chronic fibrotic sarcoidosis. Although often across the nose and cheeks, these violaceous plaques may be found on the arms, buttocks and thighs. Nasal septal perforation may occur. It is treated with prednisolone and weekly methotrexate. Sarcoidosis also has a predilection for scars and tattoos and can cause subcutaneous nodules.

94 A man, aged 58, with a 4-week history of dysphagia, presented with a short history of vomiting followed by dyspnoea and chest pain. The chest radiograph (**94**) was taken before any intervention. What does it show and what is the likely cause?

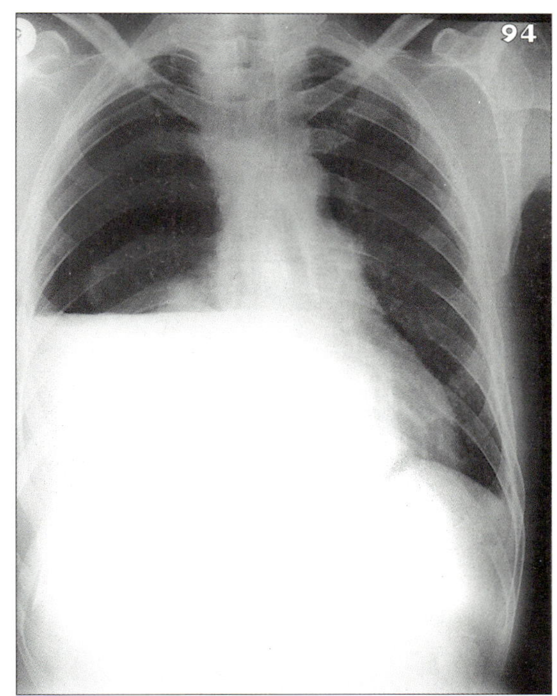

95 i. A 22-year-old girl sought advice from her general practitioner because her dormitory co-habitors complained of her snoring.
i. What is shown in **95** and what is the natural history of this condition?
ii. What is the diagnosis?
iii. How would you confirm the diagnosis?
iv. How would you treat her condition and what precaution would you take?
v. What other physical abnormalities may predispose to OSA?

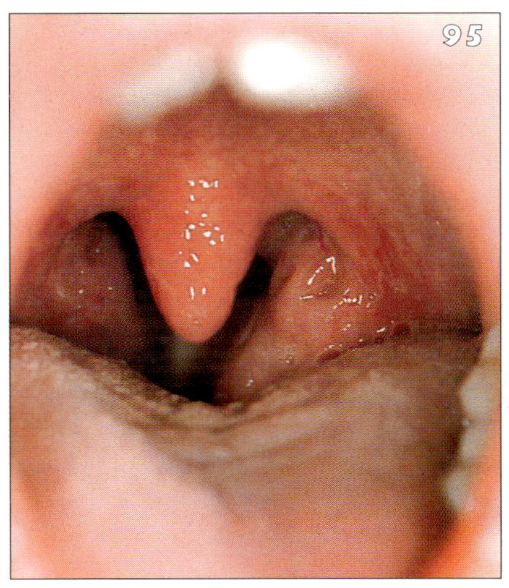

94 Hydropneumothorax. The presence of a large quantity of both air and fluid in the pleural cavity in a patient with these symptoms is strongly suggestive of rupture of the oesophagus. The fluid was turbid, but not purulent. The underlying cause was ulceration of the oesophagus by tuberculous mediastinal lymph nodes. Rupture of the oesophagus can occur in previously fit individuals, for example after violent vomiting or impaction of food bolus or foreign body, and is a medical emergency. It initially may cause retrosternal or pleural pain. It may be missed at oesophagoscopy if the tear is small, and is best diagnosed by a barium swallow. Immediate repair by a thoracic surgeon is the treatment of choice. Rupture can also occur as a result of an oesophageal tumour causing necrosis of the wall. This may also occur with tracheal tumour or metastatic subcarinal nodes. Ensleevement of the lesion with an oesophageal tube can give good palliation. Other possible causes of hydropneumothorax include rupture of a large lung abscess, empyema or rupture of a tuberculous cavity into the pleural space. Simple aspiration would be inadequate and drainage with a large-bore intercostal tube is mandatory, together with appropriate intravenous antibiotic therapy.

95 i. Enlarged tonsils. In adults, tonsils normally atrophy but some individuals with persistently enlarged tonsils can develop obstructive sleep apnoea.
ii. Obstructive sleep apnoea due to large tonsils.
iii. Sleep study. Polysomnography is considered the gold-standard for the diagnosis of OSA. Other limited or partial sleep studies which are also used include the following:
- Pulse oximetry alone to measure arterial oxygen desaturation (specificity 100%, sensitivity 31%).
- Pulse oximetry + measurement of respiratory effort + body position + snoring + measurement of sleep fragmentation.

Respiratory effort can be measured by a video-camera recording, assessing irregularities in the thoracoabdominal movement (phase-angle paradox) by inductance plethysmography or by measuring airflow limitation.
iv. Tonsillectomy. If the OSA is severe, the patient should be on nasal CPAP immediately after surgery because anaesthesia, opiates and pharyngeal oedema/haematoma may aggravate OSA postoperatively.
v. The physical signs to look out for are: those that can cause OSA such as obesity, nasal obstruction, significant overcrowding of teeth, micrognathia, retrognathia, a swollen and oedematous palate, oedematous and swollen pharynx with redundant folds, tonsils, large tongue, large neck circumference, inspiratory snore or snort even when awake, hypothyroid facies, acromegalic facies, spider naevi and alcoholic breath.

96 Shown (**96a**) is a high-power photomicrograph of a Gram stain of expectorated sputum produced by a 68-year-old man with steroid-dependent COPD. He had symptoms of fatigue, weight loss and pleuritic chest pain of 5 weeks' duration. A chest radiograph showed a cavitary left upper lobe infiltrate extending to the pleural surface.

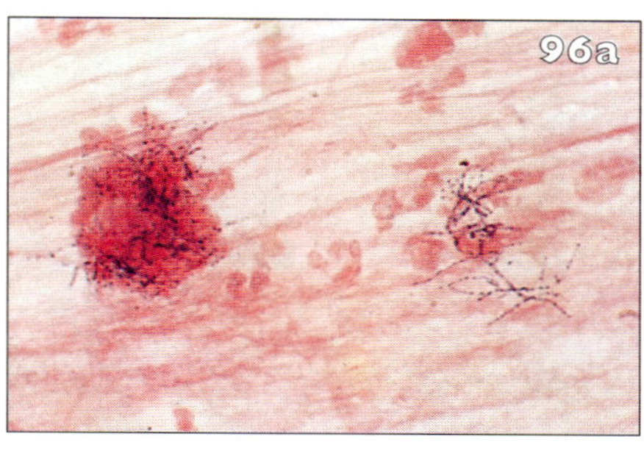

i. What is seen on the Gram stain (**96a**)?
ii. What is the differential diagnosis of the clinical and microbiological findings?
iii. What are the relevant diagnostic and therapeutic considerations?

97 The peak flow chart shown in **97** was recorded by a spray painter who worked from 9 am to 5 pm, Monday to Friday. His symptoms were often worse at night.
i. Is this consistent with occupational asthma?
ii. Why is there peak flow improvement during the first few hours at work?

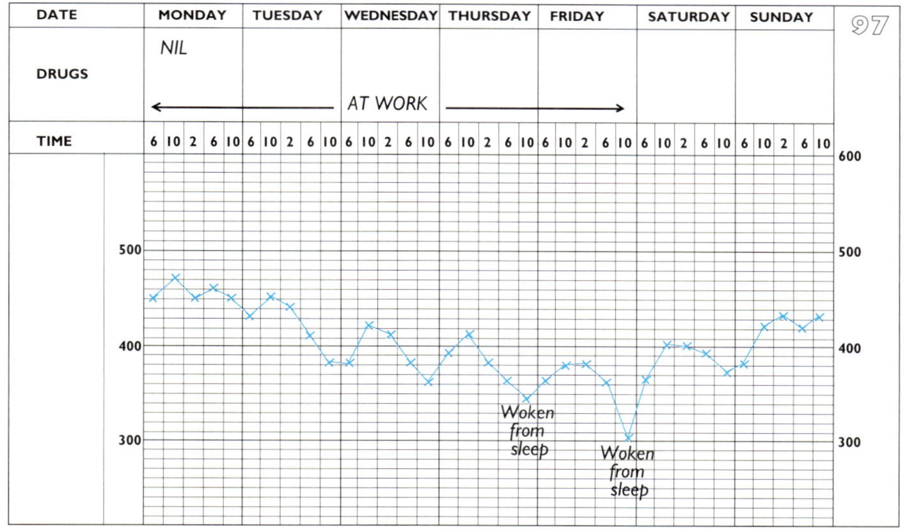

96 i. The Gram-stained specimen contains numerous polymorphonuclear leukocytes, strands of mucous, and clumps of beaded, branching Gram-positive rods.
ii. The Gram stain suggests either *Nocardia* or *Actinomyces* species.
iii. Either can produce an insidious or subacute pulmonary infection, mimicking fungal or mycobacterial infection, or malignancy. Actinomycosis occurs more often in men with periodontal or underlying lung disease, and may progress to chest wall invasion and sinus tract formation. Direct invasion of thoracic viscera and systemic dissemination are possible. Yellow 'sulphur granules' in the draining pus are virtually diagnostic of actinomycosis. However, isolation of *Actinomyces* from the respiratory tract is non-specific because the organism can exist as a commensal oropharyngeal colonizer. Definitive diagnosis requires isolation from a sterile site or histological demonstration of tissue invasion. Nocardiosis occurs more commonly in immunocompromised patients and has a greater propensity to disseminate, especially to the brain. Because *Nocardia* are rarely isolated in the absence of clinical disease, a positive culture is usually considered diagnostic. *Nocardia* are often weakly acid-fast

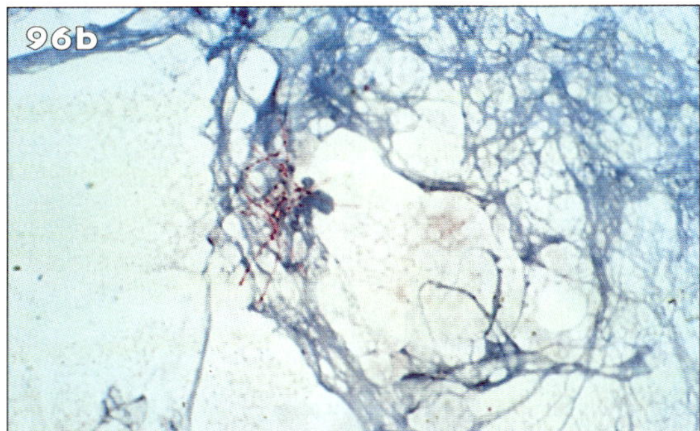

when stained with the modified Ziehl–Neelsen method (**96b**). Actinomycosis should be treated with a prolonged course of penicillin, whereas prolonged treatment with trimethoprim/ sulphamethoxazole is recommended for nocardiosis. Surgical drainage is necessary for management of abscess or empyema.

97 i. There are many patterns of occupational asthma; this pattern is one of the more common and shows a decline in peak flows as the week progresses, with worsening at night after leaving work and variable improvement at the week-end. Isocyanate in the paint was the likely cause in this case as the reaction and drop in peak flow is often delayed. Other patterns of occupational asthma include development of symptoms within minutes of arriving at work or, more chronically, sometimes fixed airflow obstruction which gradually improves only after weeks away from work. Recovery from asthma due to isocyanate may be very slow, particularly in cases of chronic exposure. Patients may remain asthmatic after removal from the offending agent.
ii. In occupational asthma, as with other forms of the condition, peak flows are often at their lowest on waking so that by mid-morning there may be an apparent improvement despite the patient being at work. This phenomenon may also affect peak flow records performed at unusual hours of the day in shift workers.

98 A cytological specimen (98) is taken from a lymph node of a HIV-positive homosexual Caucasian patient who has a CD4 count of 0.02×10^9/l, complains of intermittent fevers and weight loss, and has developed anaemia and lymphadenopathy.

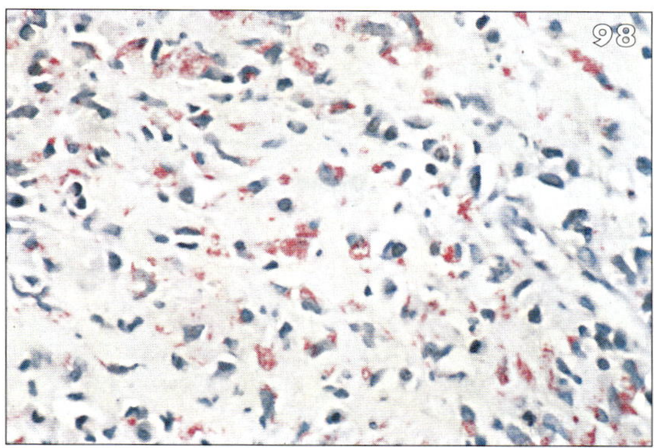

i. What is the diagnosis?
ii. How may this condition affect the lung?
iii. What are the treatment options?

99 The hypnograms (99) reflect a computerized summary of the sleep stages in an individual with obstructive sleep apnoea (OSA) before (top trace) and immediately after (bottom trace) beginning therapy with nasal continuous positive airway pressure (CPAP). REM sleep (highlighted in blue) and sleep stages (1, 2, 3, 4) are shown.
i. The durations of which sleep stages are increased by initiation of CPAP?
ii. What are the potential consequences of this?
iii. What are the effects of benzodiazepines, tricyclic antidepressants and alcohol on the hypnogram?

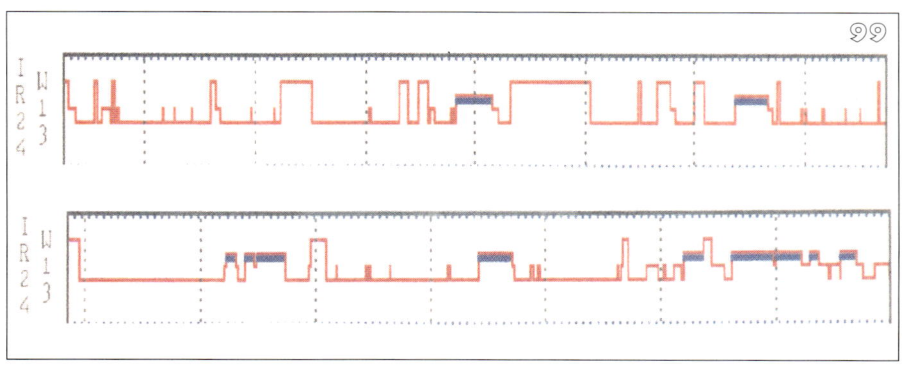

98 i. The slide shows mycobacteria (pink staining). In view of the history (very low CD4 count, typical clinical history and lack of risk factors for tuberculosis) this is most likely to be atypical mycobacteriosis – most usually organisms of the *Mycobacterium avium–intracellulare* complex (MAC). However, such a patient should be treated as tuberculosis until the bacterial cultures prove otherwise.
ii. Pulmonary involvement can occur during MAC infection although other atypical mycobacteria (e.g. *M. kansasii*) are more likely to be detected in primary lung disease. The presenting features of pulmonary disease due to atypical mycobacteria are similar to HIV-related tuberculosis, although as these organisms normally only cause disease at very low CD4 lymphocyte counts ($<0.1\times10^9$/l). Non-specific interstitial shadowing and hilar/mediastinal adenopathy are the most common features.
iii. *In vitro* antibiotic sensitivity patterns are less helpful for these organisms than for *M. tuberculosis* in that with MAC in particular, antibiotics to which the organism shows *in vitro* resistance often show clinical efficacy. Combinations of rifampicin or rifabutin and ethambutol with clarithromycin and clofazamine often bring about a short-term remission. If fever and other systemic features do not respond to antibiotics, oral steroids can bring about symptomatic relief in what is likely to be a patient with a poor prognosis.

99 i. Sleep apnoea syndromes may be associated with suppression of slow wave (Stages 3 and 4) and rapid eye movement (REM) sleep. REM suppression is more common in adults, in contrast to the predominance of slow wave suppression in children. On initiation of CPAP, there is a large rebound of slow wave and REM sleep which is most marked during the first night and which lasts about a week.
ii. There is a marked depression of arousability and unusually long and intense REM episodes occur. Sleep-disordered breathing tends to be more frequent and severe during REM sleep, and patients may become susceptible to hypoxaemia as a result of this. Patients with severe sleep apnoea who are treated with inadequate CPAP pressures may be especially at risk of severe hypoxaemia. For this reason, some experts recommend that such patients be treated for the first night under close supervision.
iii. Benzodiazepines tend to suppress slow wave sleep but do not affect REM sleep. Tricyclic antidepressants and alcohol tend to suppress REM sleep. Withdrawal from a drug which tends to suppress a stage of sleep is usually associated with a rebound of that stage. For example, as alcohol is metabolized there is often a rebound of REM sleep after an initial period of suppression.

100 This patient presented with breathlessness and reticulonodular shadowing on chest radiograph (**100**) suggestive of cryogenic fibrosing alveolitis. A transbronchial biopsy was negative. List the arguments for and against open lung biopsy.

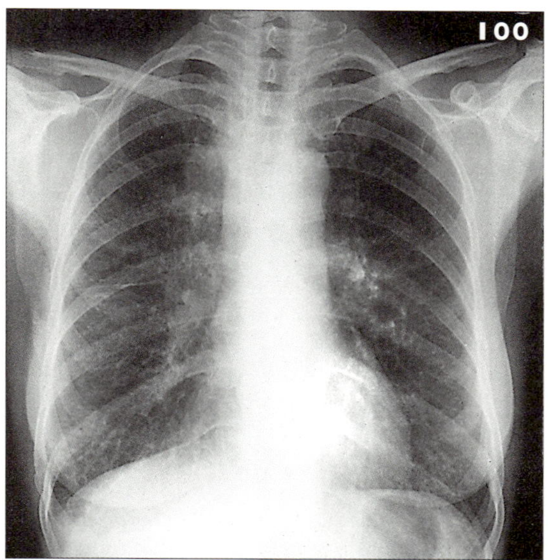

101 Shown (**101**) is the chest radiograph of a 22-year-old man resuscitated in the emergency department and treated for a presumed diagnosis of pulmonary oedema. Shortly after admission to ITU a pulmonary artery catheter was placed and the following haemodynamic data obtained 2 hours after his arrival in the emergency department (pressures in mmHg measured from sternal angle with patient semi-recumbent): RAP, –1;

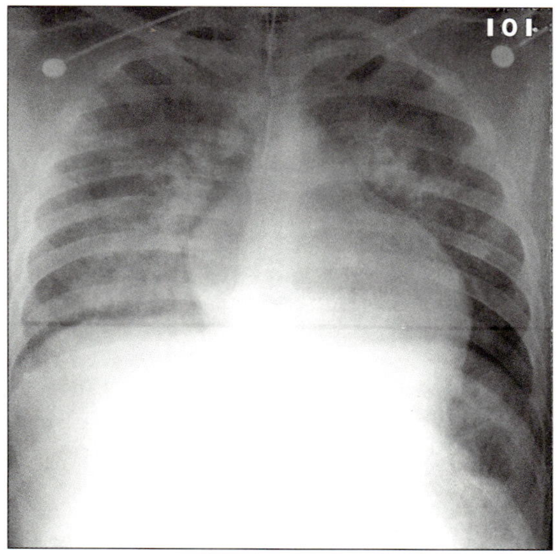

mean PAP, +12; PAOP, +8; systemic arterial pressure, 105/75, mean MAP, 83; heart rate:,100; cardiac output (Q), 4 l/min.

i. What does the chest radiograph (**100**) show and how do you interpret the PA catheter findings?

ii. What other investigations would be of relevance?

100 Arguments for:
- Open lung biopsy allows analysis of a greater quantity of alveolar tissue and strengthens the chance of detecting a range of fibrosis intensities. At least two biopsies should be taken from lung regions which appear different in terms of disease effect.
- In cases where transbronchial biopsy has not made an alternative diagnosis such as sarcoidosis or lymphangitis carcinomatosa, an open lung biopsy can rule these out with certainty.
- Histology which is predominantly cellular may persuade the physician to persist longer with anti-inflammatory therapy.
- It may allow for analysis of metals and silicates in cases where an occupational cause is suspected.

Arguments against:
- Most clinicians still give a trial of steroids regardless of whether the biopsy is predominantly cellular or fibrotic as response to therapy is not always predicted by the biopsy.
- OLB is often performed in patients who are severely compromised in terms of gas exchange. The added trauma of the procedure may result in the patient requiring prolonged positive-pressure ventilation. Complications include persistent air leak, empyema and haemorrhage. Mortality may be as high as 5%.
- High-resolution CT scans provide high-quality images which allow the diagnosis to be made with reasonable certainty.

101 i. The chest radiograph (**101**) shows a globular and enlarged heart (although AP film makes precise quantification inappropriate) and widespread alveolar infiltrates. The patient has been intubated. The appearances would be consistent with (cardiogenic) pulmonary oedema, atypical pneumonia or acute respiratory distress syndrome (ARDS).

The systemic and pulmonary vascular resistances (SVR, PVR) calculated in Wood units (mmHg/l/min) from the catheter data are:
- SVR = (MAP – RAP)/ Q = 21
- PVR = (PAP – PAOP)/ Q = 1

The SVR is raised (normal 18) and the PVR is normal, which would be unusual both for severe pneumonia/sepsis and ARDS. The PAOP is only mildly elevated and this would appear to exclude cardiogenic pulmonary oedema.

ii. It is **not** possible to differentiate between cardiogenic pulmonary oedema, atypical pneumonia and ARDS on chest radiographic appearances alone, since all produce an increase in interstitial lung water and, with increasing severity, alveolar flooding. The history of the onset of the acute illness, relevant past medical history, clinical signs, drug therapy and the results and timing of subsequent investigations are necessary information to distinguish between these conditions.

102 A patient complained of coughing with drinking and had a past history of hiatus hernia repair in infancy with subsequent oesophageal stricture formation and multiple dilatations.

i. What examination (**102**) has been performed and what does it reveal?

ii. What is the likely mechanism for this process?

iii. What other more common condition can cause this problem and where would the lesion typically be located?

iv. What are the therapeutic options?

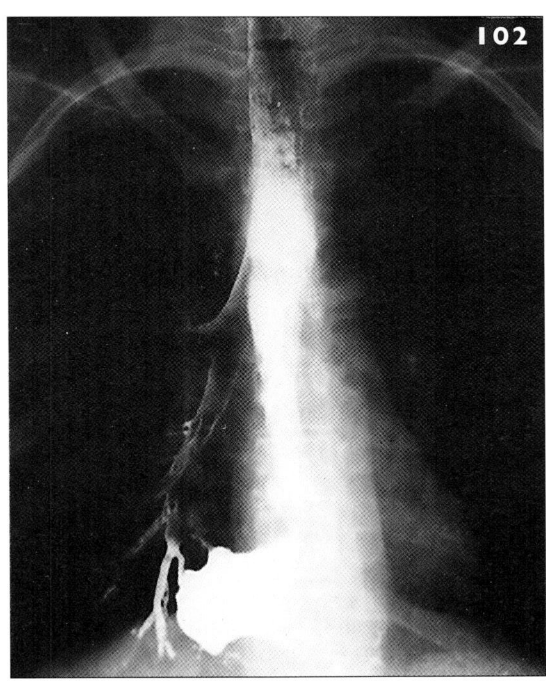

103 Shown (**103**) is the chest radiograph of a 44-year-old man with a non-productive cough for 3 months that resolved after treatment for post-nasal drip. Skin tests were negative for tuberculin and positive for histoplasmin. He recalled no childhood respiratory illnesses and had been raised on a farm in Illinois.

i. What are the radiographic findings?

ii. What is the differential diagnosis?

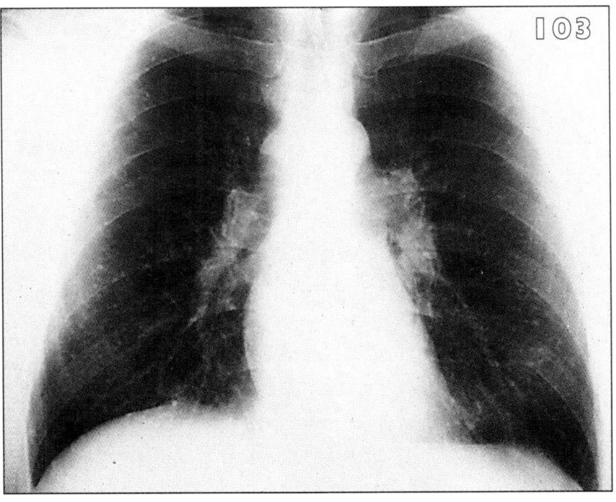

102 i. This is a barium swallow that shows an oesophagobronchial fistula. There is a distal oesophageal stricture with a right paraoesophageal abscess cavity communicating with the oesophagus and the lower right bronchial system.
ii. It is likely that the distal oesophagus was perforated at a dilatation attempt. This has resulted in the paraoesophageal abscess cavity which has eroded into the right bronchial tree.
iii. More commonly this problem results from an oesophageal carcinoma involving the trachea or proximal left main bronchus. This is particularly likely to result from radiotherapy for an advanced oesophageal tumour. Erosion of a proximal bronchogenic carcinoma into the oesophagus is also possible, but less frequent.
iv. In this case, an unusual situation, right thoracotomy to disconnect the lung from the paraoesophageal abscess cavity would be necessary. The oesophagus would have to be repaired and the stricture corrected. Chronic inflammatory changes can make surgery in this situation very difficult. For an oesophagotracheal fistula due to tumour, an endoprosthesis or sheathed stent offers the best prospect for both relieving obstruction (usually oesophageal) and occluding the fistula.

103 i. The chest radiograph (**103**) shows hilar and paratracheal adenopathy, and diffusely scattered, small, calcified, parenchymal lung nodules. This appearance suggests a remote, and now 'healed' disseminated infection.
ii. The differential diagnosis includes previous infections (e.g. Varicella or histoplasmosis) or, less likely, sarcoidosis. Miliary tuberculosis or disseminated coccidioidomycosis are unlikely to have resolved spontaneously, and transbronchial lung biopsies failed to demonstrate active peribronchial granulomatous inflammation. Thus, 'old' histoplasmosis is the most likely explanation for this patient's radiographic abnormalities. Histoplasmosis results from the inhalation of spores of the dimorphic soil fungus, *Histoplasma capsulatum*, which is endemic to the central river valleys of North America. Acute infection is often asymptomatic but occasionally can result in a pneumonia-like illness or even the acute respiratory distress syndrome. Parenchymal infiltrates and hilar adenopathy may be seen even in asymptomatic patients. Fibrosis and calcification often accompany resolution of these infections, and hepatosplenic calcification may also be present. Most patients recover without medical intervention. Some patients (generally those with underlying lung disease) fail to clear the initial infection and develop chronic pulmonary histoplasmosis which clinically and radiologically resembles tuberculosis. Progressive disseminated histoplasmosis can be life-threatening, especially in patients with defective cell-mediated immunity. This may occur during progressive primary infection but more often results from reactivation in previously infected patients. Both chronic and disseminated histoplasmosis should be treated with amphotericin B, although oral itraconazole may be used in milder cases. Immunocompromised patients require chronic suppressive itraconazole therapy.

104 A colleague asks for assistance interpreting the lung volumes measured in the patient with radiograph in **104**. The total lung capacity measured by helium dilution was 83% predicted and the residual volume was 95% predicted.
i. How can you explain the normal TLC and RV?
ii. What test would you recommend?

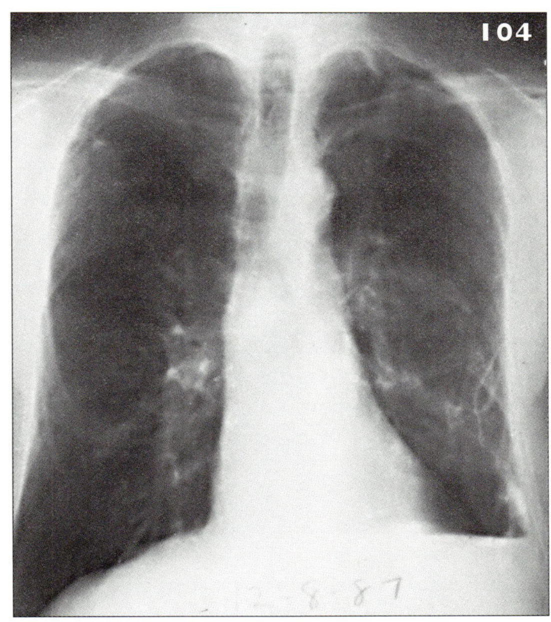

105 i. What process is being performed here (**105**)?
ii. What is the most common acute respiratory illness associated with this process?
iii. What are the causal agents and underlying pathophysiology?

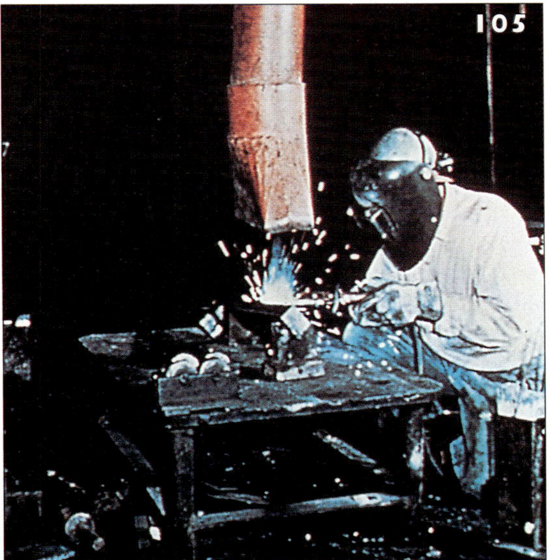

104 i. The total lung capacity (TLC) and the residual volume appear falsely low because the radiograph shown suggests larger than normal lung volumes with flat diaphragms. This is a common problem when the helium dilution technique or any other inert gas technique is used to measure lung volumes in the presence of severe airflow obstruction or bullous lung disease. This is because the test does not allow sufficient re-breathing or washout time for the inert gas to enter the poorly ventilated areas of the lung. Thus, there is often a gross under-estimation of the true lung volume. Gas dilution techniques are, however, quite accurate when used in normal subjects or patients without airflow obstruction.

ii. Repeating the measurement of lung volumes using a body plethysmograph will provide much more accurate estimates in patients with airway problems and emphysema. The method has the advantage that it measures the total volume of gas in the lung, including any that is trapped behind closed airways which are not communicating easily with the mouth. Plethysmography is, therefore, the technique of choice in patients with airflow obstruction.

105 i. Electric arc welding using a manual system remains widespread, despite automation, and requires the worker to be close to the work piece and accompanying welding plume. Local exhaust ventilation (present in this instance) and the use of an appropriate mask respirator limit the worker's exposure to fumes.

ii. Metal fume fever. This self-limited illness resembling influenza afflicts most career welders at least once during their lifetime. A mild pharyngitis and cough may be present during the exposure. Constitutional symptoms are delayed 4–8 h after the initial exposure and consist of fevers to 41°C, myalgia, malaise, nausea, headache and cough. Complete resolution occurs within 24–48 h after exposure. Therapy is limited to antipyretics and mild analgesics.

iii. Zinc oxide fumes are the most common cause of metal fume fever. Fumes of copper, magnesium and, less commonly, aluminium, cadmium, chromium, nickel and tin are also associated with metal fume fever. Repeated exposure to fumes produces tolerance to the illness which is rapidly lost with time away from work. This phenomenon produces 'Monday morning fever', a well-recognized presentation among welders.

106 Shown (**106**) is a photomicrograph of PAS-stained lung tissue obtained at autopsy from a 41-year-old man with AIDS who presented initially with dyspnoea, cough, malaise and fever. An induced sputum specimen suggested the diagnosis of *P. carinii* pneumonia, but he deteriorated and died despite treatment.

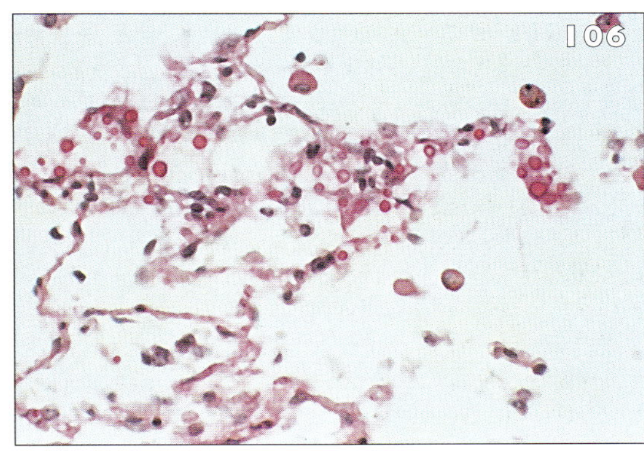

i. What diagnosis is suggested by the histological findings?
ii. How could this diagnosis be confirmed?
iii. What is the appropriate treatment?

107 These radiographs (**107a, 107b**) are from a patient who has undergone laser resection of a tumour occluding the left main bronchus.
i. What has happened?
ii. What predictive factors are there for this occurring?

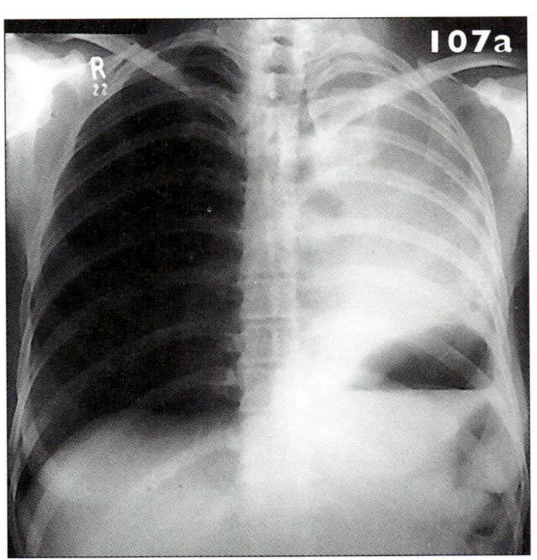

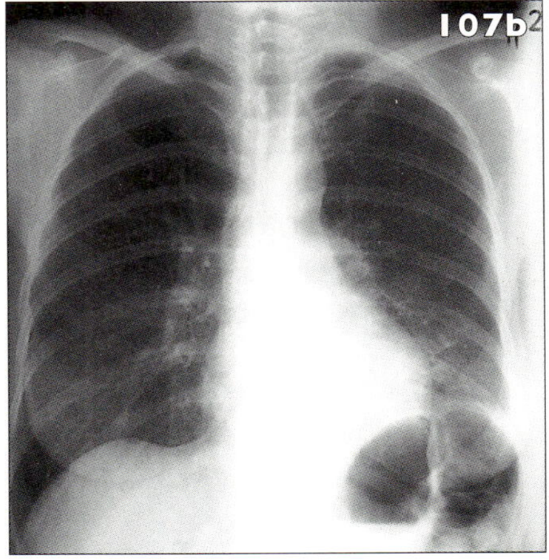

106 i. The histology shows alveolar tissue with minimal inflammatory changes but numerous, pink-staining yeast forms with varying degrees of encapsulation. A fungal culture of the lung tissue grew *C. neoformans*. Cryptococci are encapsulated yeasts with a worldwide distribution. As with the geographic fungi, it is a soil organism which flourishes in areas enriched by sources of organic nitrogen (e.g. bird droppings) and is acquired by inhalation. A thick capsule inhibits phagocytosis by neutrophils, although virulent acapsular strains exist. A cell-mediated immune response is necessary to contain cryptococcal infection. Asymptomatic pulmonary infection is common and spontaneous resolution is the rule in normal hosts. Patients with defects in cell-mediated immunity can develop progressive lung involvement. Extrapulmonary spread is common, especially to the meninges.
ii. The diagnosis of cryptococcosis is complicated by the fact that the organisms can colonize the upper airway and contaminate cultures of respiratory secretions. The chest radiograph may show a single mass, multiple nodules, or infiltrates with associated hilar adenopathy. Encapsulated yeasts invading the tissue are easily seen using routine histological stains. Finally, cryptococcal antigen can rapidly be identified in the blood of most patients with pneumonia and in the CSF of nearly all with meningitis.
iii. No treatment is necessary for cryptococcal pneumonia in an immunocompetent host without meningitis. Aggressive antifungal therapy with amphotericin B and flucytosine is indicated for all patients with meningitis and for immunocompromised patients with isolated respiratory infection. Immunocompromised patients require chronic suppressive oral therapy.

107 i. There has been re-expansion of a totally collapsed lung due to removal of the endobronchial part of the tumour. Improved breathlessness and lung function occur and improved ventilation and perfusion of the previously collapsed lung can be demonstrated by radionuclide scans. It may also permit drainage of infected retained secretions.
ii. It is difficult to predict which patients will have such improvement. Where a tumour has progressed radiographically from the periphery towards the hilum the obstruction is unlikely to respond to removal of the proximal part of the tumour by laser. Shorter duration of collapse (up to 3 months) is more likely to respond to attempts at re-expansion. During the procedure it may be difficult to know how far distally an obstruction extends; a CT scan can sometimes help in this regard. An attempt should be made early in the procedure to pass through the obstruction and assess the patency of the distal airways. If these are occluded the likelihood of a favourable outcome is small.

108 The chest radiograph in **108** is from a 40-year-old patient.
i. What is the major abnormality that is seen?
ii. What is the differential diagnosis of this abnormality?

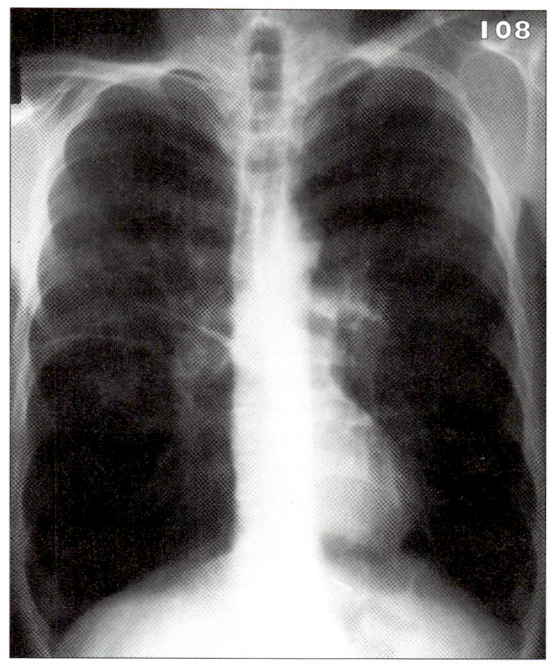

109 **i.** What operation has this patient undergone (**109**)?
ii. Why is there a scoliosis?

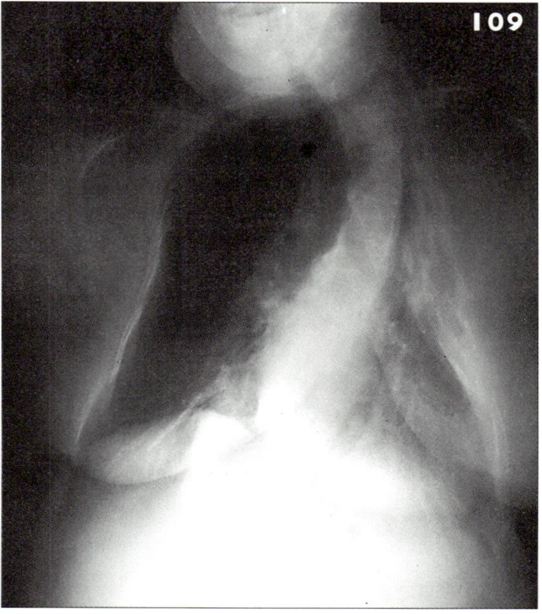

108 i. Emphysema, primarily affecting the lung bases bilaterally.
ii. Bibasilar emphysema in a relatively young patient most commonly results from α-antitrypsin deficiency. Recently, this pattern has also been described as a result of i.v. methylphenidate (Ritalin®) abuse. α-1-Antitrypsin deficiency is an inherited lack of this protease which can lead to panlobular emphysema in the third or fourth decade of life, particularly in those who smoke. Intravenous injection of Ritalin, an amphetamine-like substance, can produce panlobular emphysema indistinguishable from that caused by α-1-antitrypsin deficiency. Emphysema secondary to smoking is usually centrilobular, is more commonly apical than basilar, and typically does not cause severe airflow obstruction until patients are in their mid-60s.

The management of α-1-antitrypsin deficiency is: (a) smoking cessation; (b) attempts to optimize bronchial dilatation (usually ineffective); (c) aggressive treatment of respiratory tract infection; or (d) single lung transplantation. Replacement therapy is too expensive to be routinely available. Family members should be screened to identify heterozygotes. There is no evidence of deterioration in the lungs of heterozygotes even if they smoke.

109 i. Left thoracoplasty. The most common indication for this operation was tuberculosis in the pre-chemotherapy area to collapse the lung in the face of progressive or uncontrolled advance of the TB. Initially the patient would have been treated by an artificial prierothorax, often for up to 1 or 2 years – also reducing the aerobic environment the *M. tuberculosis* organism enjoys. It was performed in 1–3 stages developed to discern the extent of patient tolerance of the procedure.

Other methods used to achieve the same result were plombage (plastic spheres inserted extra-pleurally inside the chest) and oleothorax (installation of paraffin wax). Thoracoplasty may rarely be performed now in patients who have chronic lung cavities with ongoing systemic symptoms, usually due to infection by resistant organisms, or in patent pleural spaces with failure of the lung to expand and fill the space.
ii. Scoliosis can develop after thoracoplasty in pre-pubertal patients and its severity was related to the number of ribs removed. The scoliosis is convex to the side of the surgery. Spinal tuberculosis may also have been a concomitant feature in such patients.

Patients with this type of chest wall deformity are at risk of nocturnal hypoventilation, particularly when there is accompanying chronic obstructive airways disease (many of these patients continue to smoke!). Ultimately, hypercapnic respiratory failure (hypoxaemia with hypercapnia) and pulmonary hypertension develop requiring oxygen therapy at night and non-invasive ventilatory support – often just at night.

110 This patient has had a series of lower respiratory tract infections, sometimes associated with wheezy breathlessness, particularly at night. The cause is shown on the lateral chest radiograph (**110a**).
i. What is it?
ii. What other investigations can confirm the diagnosis?

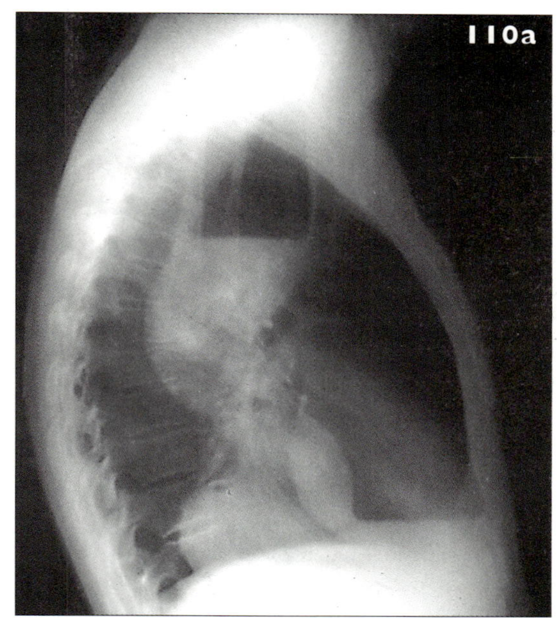

111 The pulmonary function tests (Table) were obtained on a 23-year-old, 225-kg male before a gastropexy planned for obesity.
i. What is the pulmonary function test abnormality?
ii. Does the patient have an intrapulmonary cause for a restrictive pulmonary disease (e.g. pulmonary fibrosis)?
iii. What pathophysiological processes contribute to the restrictive pattern seen?
iv. Will these tests improve with weight loss?

Function	Predicted	Best measured	% predicted
FVC (l)	6.05	3.72	61
FEV_1 (l)	4.80	3.05	64
FEV_1/FVC	0.79	0.82	104
PEFR (l/s)	–	6.10	–
$FEF_{25-75\%}$ (l/s)	4.51	3.45	76
FRC (l, BTPS)	4.15	1.42	34
RV (l, BTPS)	2.27	1.01	45
TLC (l, BTPS)	8.23	4.94	60
RV/TLC	0.27	0.20	75
DL_{CO} (ml/m/mm Hg)	47.78	29.13	61
DL_{CO}/VA	5.27	4.95	94

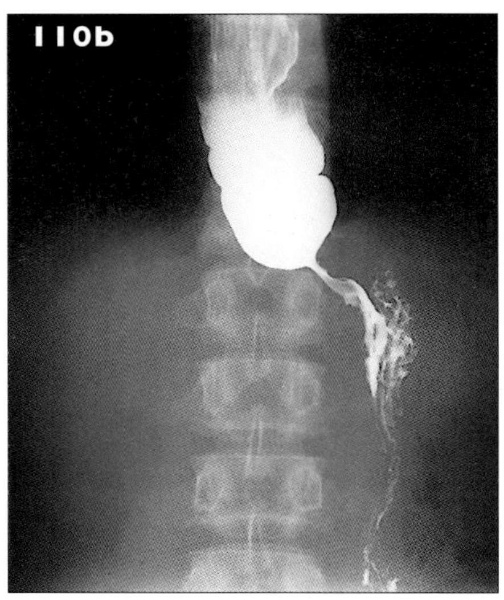

110 i. The lateral chest radiograph shows a mega-oesophagus which is tortuous within the thorax and has a clearly shown fluid level at the level of the manubrium, which also illustrates the large size the oesophagus has attained. A PA chest film may show mediastinal widening and sometimes a fluid level. The abnormality is due to chronic contraction of the lower oesophageal sphincter. Occasionally, chronic obstruction by benign or malignant disease may lead to mega-oesophagus. Sometimes these patients are treated and diagnosed as asthma.

ii. A barium swallow will confirm the diagnosis and exclude other causes of obstruction (**110b**). The condition is usually treated by oesophagoscopy and dilatation of the sphincter, but sometimes a surgical myotomy is required. The respiratory tract infections and wheezing bouts are due to aspiration of oesophageal contents into the lung, particularly when the patient lies flat.

111 i. A restrictive pattern of disease.

ii. These tests are consistent with obesity, i.e. an extrathoracic cause. Without further clinical information, no other diagnosis, including that of pulmonary fibrosis need be sought. For obesity to cause a reduced TLC the weight (in kg)/height (in cm) ratio must generally exceed 1.0. Reductions in functional residual capacity (FRC), vital capacity (VC) and residual volume (RV) can occur with lesser degrees of obesity. The reduced gas transfer (DL_{CO}) corrects to normal when alveolar volume (K_{CO}) is incorporated. This implies normal pulmonary gas exchange and the low DL_{CO} is probably due to basal hypoventilation as a direct consequence of obesity.

iii. Obese individuals have increased chest wall mass, resulting in a reduction in net outward elastic recoil pressures. Lung and chest wall compliances fall as weight increases. The increased mass of the abdominal wall and abdominal contents reduces the FRC. Accordingly, these patients develop airway closure in dependent lung zones that become most pronounced when the patient lies supine. The changes in PaO_2 observed when these patients lie supine can be great.

iv. Pulmonary function tests improve toward normal as weight is lost.

112 This patient has limited disease small-cell lung cancer (**112**).
i. What is meant by 'limited disease' and how is it staged?
ii. What is the optimal treatment?
iii. What is the likely 2- and 5-year survival?

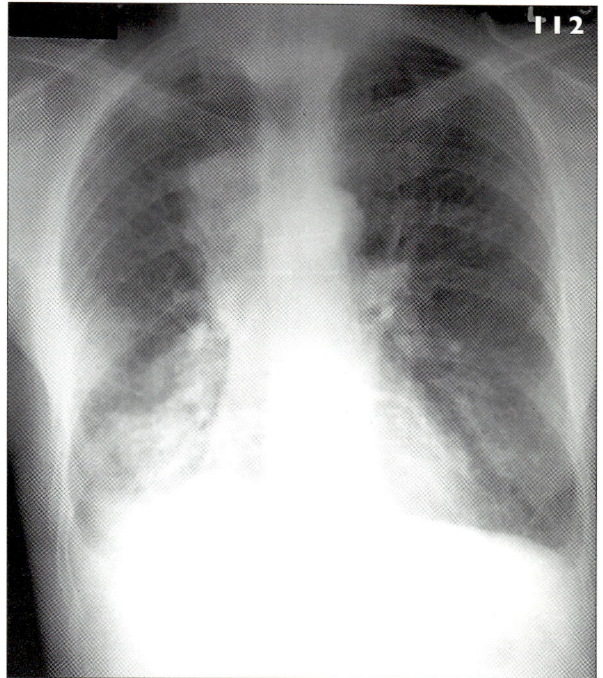

113 The data shown in the Table were obtained at maximal exercise testing in a 45-year-old man with breathlessness on exertion.
i. What does maximal oxygen uptake (VO_2max) measure and what parameters are needed to measure it?
ii. Would this patient be capable of performing a job involving packing shelves with light weight boxes?

Measurement	Observed maximum	Predicted maximum
Heart rate (beats/min)	162	160
Ventilation(l/min)	55	60
VO_2max (l/min)	1.9	–

112 i. Limited stage disease is confined to that hemithorax and the ipsilateral supraclavicular fossa. More detailed staging using the TNM system has little prognostic value, although is mandatory in the occasional SCLC that appears truly operable. The recommended staging tests for SCLC are a blood screen, a liver ultrasound and a bone scan. A CT thorax is usually unnecessary as the mediastinum often appears bulky on the plain radiography and adds little extra information.
ii. The optimal treatment is combination cytotoxic chemotherapy. Ideally, six courses should be given, one every 3 weeks. Radiotherapy to the mediastinum is recommended for patients who achieve a complete response. About 50% of patients presenting with limited disease should achieve a complete response on chest radiography and other staging tests. Radiotherapy confers a small but significant survival advantage at 2 years after the end of treatment and also reduces the incidence of relapse within the chest.
iii. The 2-year survival of limited disease of SCLC is 7%. For those patients with good prognostic variables (high performance status and normal biochemistry), then the 5-year survival is 15–20%. Of all patients alive at 2 years, 25% will still relapse with SCLC and another 20% will develop non-small-cell lung cancer within 5 years of starting treatment for SCLC.

113 i. VO_2 measures the amount of oxygen extracted by the tissues during exercise and is directly related to the amount of work performed. VO_2 = cardiac output (Q) × oxygen content difference of arterial and mixed venous blood ($CaO_2 - CvO_2$), or $VO_2 = Q \times (SaO_2 - SvO_2) \times 1.34$.

SvO_2 (the saturation of mixed venous blood) reflects the ability of the exercising muscles to extract oxygen from the blood. VO_2max is defined as the plateau of oxygen uptake where attempting to go beyond that work capacity is associated with increasing ventilation but no increase in cardiac output. This is the point where the subject has reached maximal aerobic power. Many subjects do not reach this point as it requires considerable effort and determination with unpleasant sensations of breathlessness and muscle soreness. Therefore what is often reported is the maximum VO_2 achieved and not the true VO_2max. VO_2 can be obtained from work performed on a cycle ergometer, treadmill or even stepping exercise, provided that measures of minute ventilation and mixed expired O_2 and CO_2 tensions are available.
ii. To be able to perform heavy physical labour throughout an 8-hour shift, subjects should achieve a VO_2max of >25 ml/kg/min. Subjects whose VO_2max is <15 ml/kg/min would be unable to walk at more than a normal pace. Therefore, the result here suggests he should be able to perform his relatively light tasks.

114 Shown (**114**) is the response of heart rate and ventilation to increasing oxygen uptake during a progressive work rate test in a man with alveolar proteinosis. Exercise has stopped with a heart rate at the upper limit of normal and a ventilation that was higher than normal, and the patient complained of breathlessness. The subsequent exercise test followed a procedure that improved the patient's breathlessness.
i. Comment on the two exercise test results.
ii. What was the procedure that improved the patient?

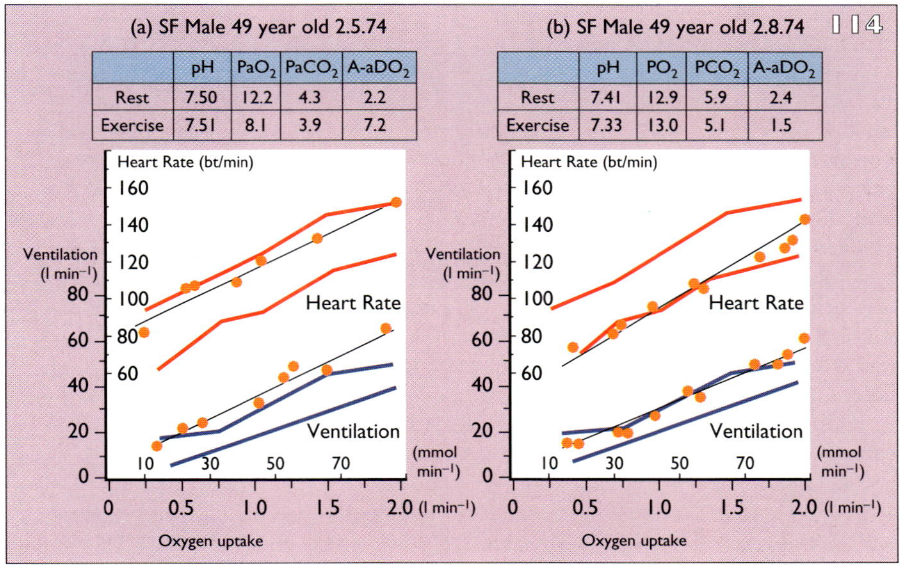

	pH	PaO₂	PaCO₂	A-aDO₂
Rest	7.50	12.2	4.3	2.2
Exercise	7.51	8.1	3.9	7.2

	pH	PO₂	PCO₂	A-aDO₂
Rest	7.41	12.9	5.9	2.4
Exercise	7.33	13.0	5.1	1.5

115 What surgical procedures might be of benefit to the patient with this CT (**115**)?

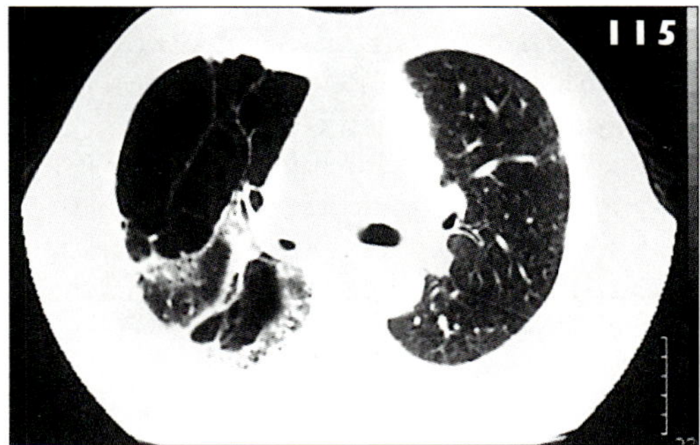

116 i. What are the usual bacterial pathogens in cystic fibrosis?
ii. How has the increase in *Burkholderia cepacia* affected clinical management?
iii. What are the clinical indications for intravenous antibiotics?

114 i. 114a shows excessively high ventilation from the beginning of exercise to the completion of the test. Arterial blood gases show hypoxaemia with increasing hypoxia at the end of exercise and a widened alveolar arterial oxygen gradient (A-aDO$_2$, 2.2 to 7.2 kPa).

The post-treatment exercise test (**114b**) shows a considerable improvement in resting heart rate and the heart rate response during exercise and the ventilatory response remained within the normal range. The arterial PO$_2$ and the alveolar arterial oxygen gradients were considerably improved.

ii. The procedure that improved the patient was a bronchoalveolar lavage of 10 l which is the treatment of choice in flushing out the abnormal protein from the alveolar spaces in these patients.

115 The patient has giant emphysematous bullae on the right with the left lung looking healthy. Removal of large bullae can result in reduction of dyspnoea and improved exercise tolerance. Two surgical techniques are available. Bullectomy is particularly indicated for the removal of a large single cyst. The operation was previously undertaken via a thoracotomy but excellent results are now being reported via the thoracoscope. The basis of the operation is to staple or suture the base of the cyst which is then excised and to fully expand the remaining lung. Nd YAG laser is also being used to perform 'lung reduction pneumoplasty'. The other option is a Monaldi-type decompression. The basis of this operation is to effect a pleurodesis so that the risk of pneumothorax is reduced and to drain individual bullae using large Foley catheters attached to underwater drainage systems. The Foley catheter balloon is inflated and the catheter is secured in the bullae by a purse string suture at the entry site. The bullae are then allowed to decompress slowly.

116 i. In an adult CF clinic the prevalence of common infecting bacterial pathogens is *P. aeruginosa* (80–90%), *Staph. aureus* (30–35%), *B. cepacia* (0–30%), *H. influenzae* (10–15%), *Str. pneumoniae* (1–3%) and *E. coli* (1%).
A. fumigatus colonizes 10–15% of patients. Its significance is uncertain.
ii. *B. cepacia* has increased in incidence and prevalence in large CF centres over the past decade. It is characterized by natural increased antibiotic resistance, greater cross-infectivity between patients, and accelerated lung disease in some patients.

Clinical management has been directed at patient segregation which has been shown to reduce the incidence and prevalence of *B. cepacia*.
iii. Intravenous antibiotics are indicated for all patients who have an infective exacerbation which is characterized by increased sputum volume, reduction in pulmonary function and weight loss.

How aggressively and frequently CF patients with relatively asymptomatic disease should be treated is uncertain. Persistently elevated serum inflammatory markers in asymptomatic patients suggests chronic progression of lung disease.

117 A patient with advanced intrathoracic squamous cell carcinoma has presented 3 weeks after completing palliative radiotherapy with confusion, vomiting and dehydration. Discuss the possible causes and management.

118 Shown are the chest radiograph (**118a**) and an abdominal CT scan (**118b**) performed 24 hours later on a 45-year-old diabetic man who had presented with abdominal pain and increasing respiratory distress.
i. What do the radiograph (**118a**) and CT scan (**118b**) show?
ii. What is the unifying diagnosis?

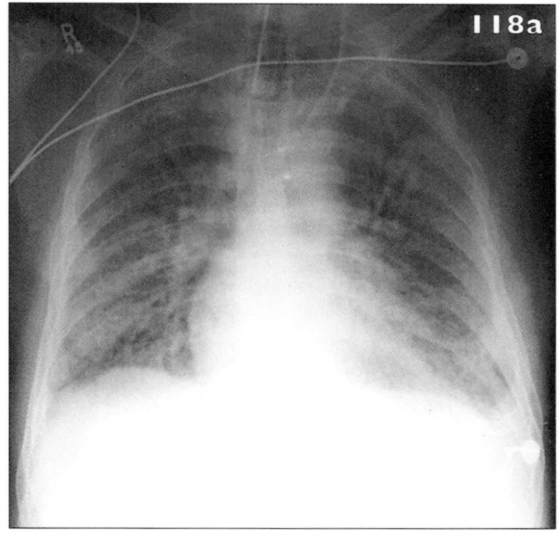

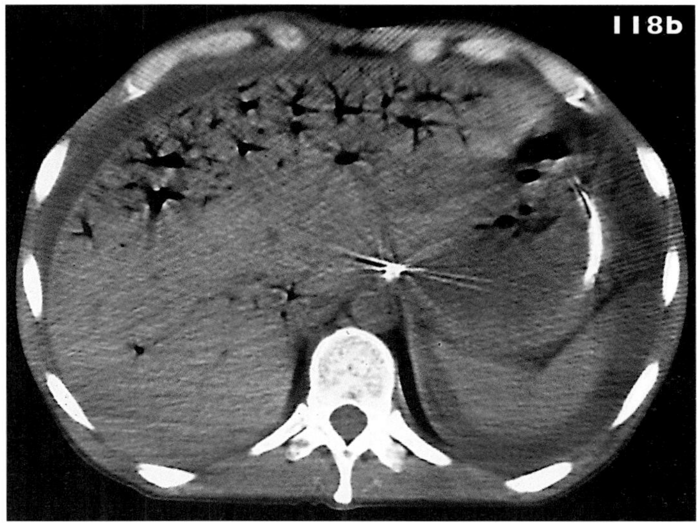

117 Possible causes include:
- Hypercalcaemia if thirst polyuria, dehydration, confusion, constipation and, ultimately, coma develop. If there is no evidence of bone pain, the likeliest cause is the primary tumour. Treatment is by rehydration, intravenous hydrocortisone and an infusion of a diphosphonate. The latter often produces dramatic effects and the benefit can last for 3–6 weeks, but may have to be repeated with either intravenous or oral diphosphonates.
- Cerebral metastasis. A CT brain scan (**117**), ideally with contrast enhancement, may show usually multiple lesions with ring enhancement from the contrast and often surrounding areas of cerebral oedema. Initial treatment is with intravenous or oral dexamethasone, 16 mg/day. If this achieves a major clinical improvement within 48 h, then whole-brain irradiation is recommended to maintain this improvement. The dexamethasone should then be rapidly reduced and stopped to reduce steroid myopathy. Should the patient not respond to 48 h of dexamethasone, then the steroids should be withdrawn and radiotherapy not offered.

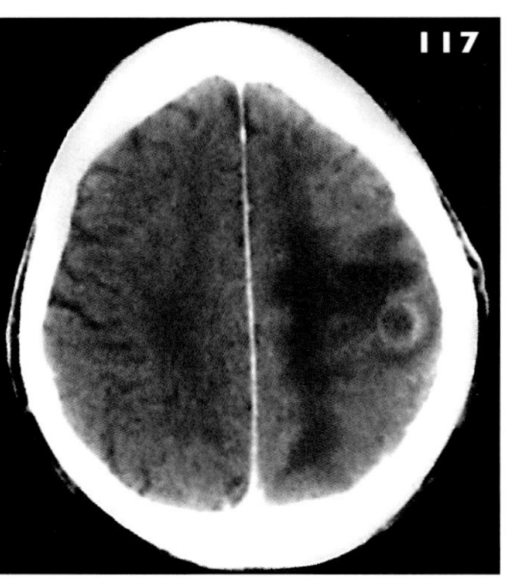

- Poor attention to analgesic treatment. The opiates and, in particular, slow-release morphine preparations can cause drowsiness and rapid dehydration and constipation. This can cause vomiting and dehydration. Opiates should always be given with a strong laxative, i.e. lactulose 20–30 ml b.d. or co-danthramer, 10–20 ml daily.

118 i. The chest radiograph (**118a**) shows that the patient is intubated and a line in the left internal jugular vein. The lung fields show widespread diffuse alveolar shadowing that would be compatible with an atypical pneumonia, acute respiratory distress syndrome and possibly pulmonary oedema. The abdominal CT scan (**118b**) shows gas in the portal venous system.
ii. The unifying diagnosis is extensive bowel necrosis leading to bowel gas and contents entering the portal venous circulation producing a severe inflammatory response with pulmonary capillary endothelial damage leading to the development of adult respiratory distress syndrome (ARDS). This clinical picture of extensive gas in the portal venous system is diagnostic of extensive bowel necrosis and is uniformly fatal.

It is important to establish the underlying cause of ARDS. ARDS is only an intermediary mechanism of disease that could be compared with jaundice or a raised RAP: the appropriate management depends on discovering the primary pathology. Management of ARDS is supportive while the underlying problem is hopefully identified and successfully treated.

119 This patient (119) had a pleural effusion aspirated 2 months previously. What is shown, what is the likely diagnosis and how might this complication have been avoided?

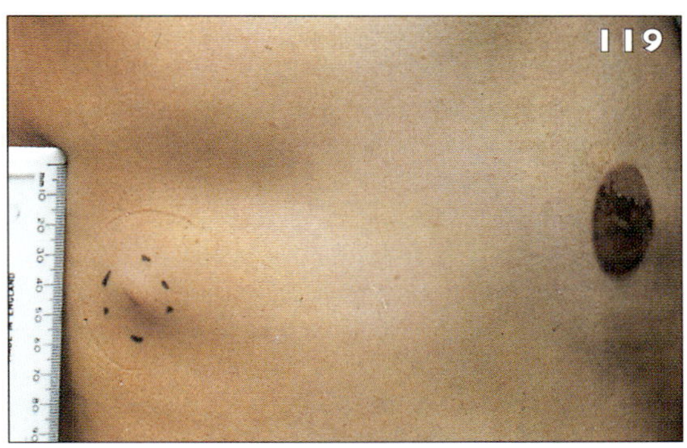

120 This 52-year-old man presented with this painless rash on his ankles (120a) and wrists (120b). The chest radiograph was abnormal.
i. Describe the rash.
ii. What pulmonary conditions are associated with this type of rash?

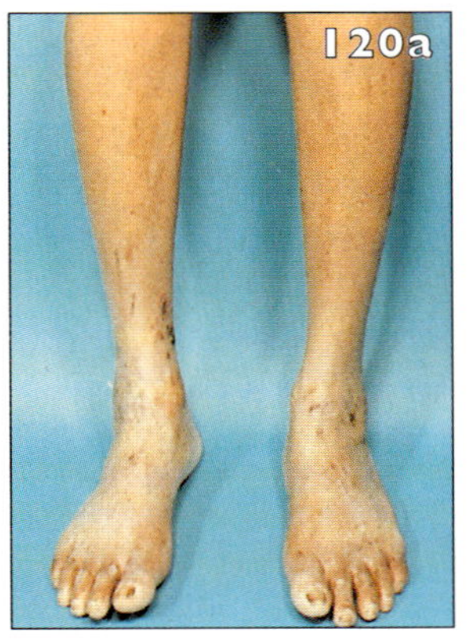

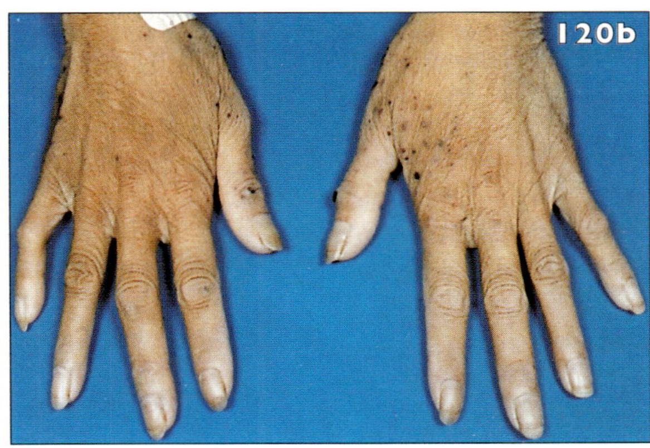

121 A 75-year-old male smoker requires surgery for bronchogenic carcinoma. His screening pulmonary function tests are: FEV_1 0.9 l (19% predicted); FVC 2.34 l (33% predicted); FEV_1/FVC 38%; TLC 7.8 l (128% predicted). His gas transfer factor (DL_{CO}) is 50% predicted with a transfer coefficient (K_{CO}) of 55% predicted.
i. Can this patient tolerate wedge resection, lobectomy or pneumonectomy?
ii. Which patients should have preoperative spirometry and/or arterial blood gas analysis before surgery?

119 Subcutaneous tumour nodule due to malignant pleural mesothelioma. Tumour seeding to the skin following aspiration, needle biopsy or surgical incision is a common complication of this condition and also of pleural adenocarcinoma, occurring in up to 50% of cases. The nodules may grow to a considerable size and cause discomfort and distress. This phenomenon can be prevented by prophylactic irradiation of needle biopsy and aspiration sites and it is therefore important to mark these sites indelibly in patients where mesothelioma is a possible diagnosis. 21 Gy, given in three fractions, is effective. Tumour seeding of this sort is much less common in malignant pleural effusion due to metastatic carcinoma or carcinoma of the bronchus.

120 i. The patient has a typical vasculitic rash with small haemorrhagic lesions on the forearms and shins.
ii. Vasculitis can affect the lungs as part of a systemic condition. The more common conditions include:
- Wegener's granulomatosis – see **152**.
- Allergic granulomatosis and angiitis (Churg–Strauss syndrome). This comprises asthma, hypereosinophilia with eosinophilic infiltrates, vasculitis and granulomata in various organs. It can be controlled by oral steroids, but the vasculitis can be life-threatening. The condition usually begins with asthma, at about 35 years of age, is of equal sex incidence, and vasculitis follows some years later. Upper airway lesions are common usually as allergic rhinitis. The ANCA test is positive in 50% of patients – predominantly p-ANCA.
- Polyarteritis nodosa (PAN) – affects medium-sized arteries, while Churg–Strauss affects small ones. There is usually no history of allergic illness in PAN and pulmonary involvement is not common. Pulmonary involvement includes asthma, pulmonary infiltrates, fibrosis and effusions. The c-ANCA test is negative.

121 i. The patient has severe airflow limitation and is not a candidate for any type of resectional surgery.
ii. Patients undergoing pulmonary resection should have pulmonary function tests to measure vital capacity, FEV_1, airflow limitation and an assessment of ventilatory capacity, such as the maximal voluntary ventilation (MVV) for 15 or 30 s, and also their CO gas transfer. Arterial blood gas tensions can generally be reserved for patients with at least moderately severe airflow limitation unless other findings suggest the possibility of hypoxaemia and/or hypercapnia. An FEV_1, FVC and MVV >55% of the predicted value are generally considered sufficient for pneumonectomy. Lobectomies can generally be tolerated with preoperative values >40%. A predicted postoperative FEV_1 of 0.8 l has traditionally been used as the lower limit of resectability (in patients of average height) based on the observations of activity level. CO_2 retention is likely to occur with lower levels of postoperative lung function. A DL_{CO} of <50% of normal is another contraindication to pulmonary resection.

122 This patient with CF presented with haemoptysis of 300–400 ml/day. He was very breathless with this due to poor underlying lung function.
i. What procedure (**122**) is being performed?
ii. What are the causes of haemoptysis in CF?

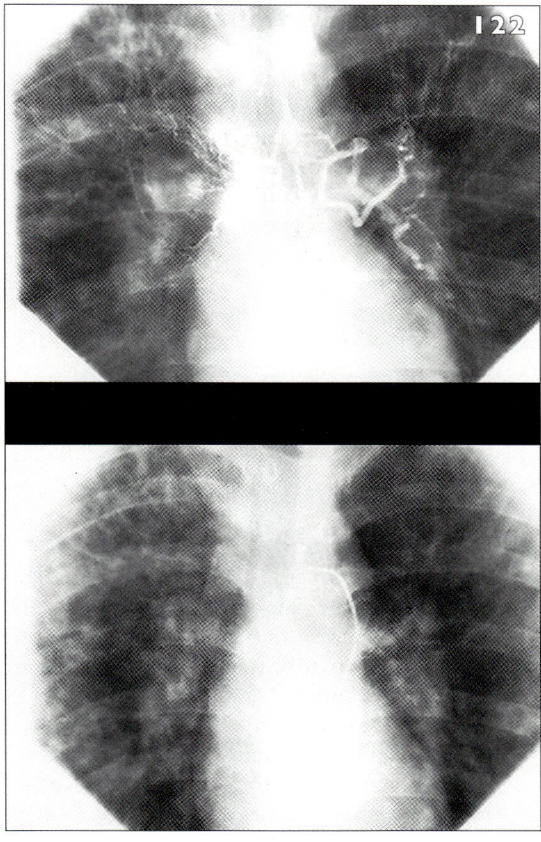

123 i. What is the device in **123**?
ii. What are its advantages and indications for use?
iii. What are its complications?

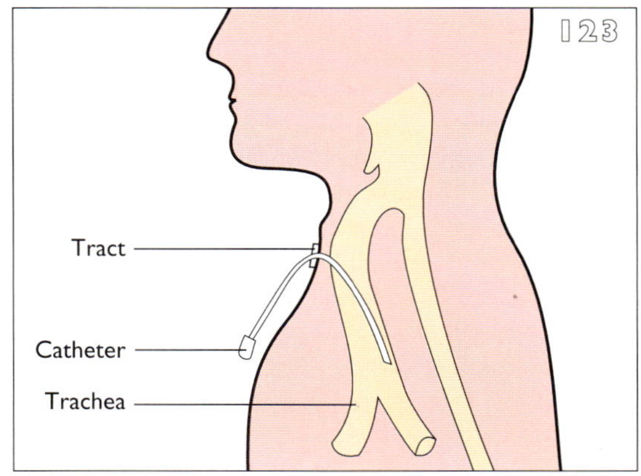

122 i. The procedure is bronchial artery angiography and embolization. The upper illustration shows a single common bronchial trunk and a flush of hypervascular vessels in the left upper lobe. There is bronchiectasis in the right upper lobe. The lower illustration shows the result following embolization of the left upper lobe vessels with PVA, a fine particulate material. The hypervascularity has been corrected, and there was complete cessation of haemoptysis. Other materials used include gel foam and small metal coils. The aim is to occlude small vessels, as occluding the larger aberrant trunk often results in opening of collateral channels.
ii. Haemoptysis is common in CF, particularly in older patients and usually only requires reassurance. Small haemoptyses (10–20 ml) usually settle with a course of antibiotics. The usual cause is rupture of small mucosal vessels where the mucosa is ulcerated and fissured due to chronic infection. Repeated coughing will aggravate haemoptysis. Contributing factors include reduced platelet count (hypersplenism) and vitamin K deficiency (liver dysfunction). Large haemoptyses (>300 ml over 24 hours) may cause severe breathlessness and be life-threatening, although this is a very unusual scenario. Intravenous pitressin is a useful holding manoeuvre. Where a bleeding bronchial artery has been demonstrated the treatment of choice is bronchial artery embolization. Surgical resection may be required in extreme cases.

123 i. The device pictured is a transtracheal catheter for the delivery of oxygen. The catheter may be positioned to exit through the skin directly overlying the trachea or may be tunnelled under the skin of the anterior chest wall to exit over the abdomen.
ii. The advantages of transtracheal oxygen delivery (compared with nasal cannulae and face masks) include:
- Improved comfort.
- Improved cosmetic appearance. An approximate 50% reduction in oxygen requirements which allows for extended delivery of oxygen from cylinders and liquid containers and increased patient mobility.
- Reduced dead space, thereby reducing ventilation and improving exercise tolerance.

Transtracheal oxygen therapy is indicated for individuals with stable chronic lung disease requiring prolonged oxygen therapy in the following situations:
- Reluctance to utilize nasal or mask oxygen therapy because of cosmetic concerns.
- Poor compliance with nasal or mask oxygen therapy because of discomfort.
- High O_2 flow rates are required to maintain adequate O_2 saturation such that routine delivery methods are not sufficient or produce excessive drying of the upper airways.

iii. Insertion of a transtracheal oxygen catheter requires local (for percutaneous catheters exiting in the neck) or general anaesthesia (for tunnelled catheters exiting elsewhere). The catheters must be removed or flushed twice daily to maintain patency. The most common complication is obstruction of the catheter by mucus plugs. On occasion these plugs can enlarge to obstruct the trachea itself.

124 Shown (**124**) is gallium-67 scan of a patient with sarcoidosis.
i. What features are physiological and pathological?
ii. What is the role of the gallium scan in sarcoidosis?
iii. Does it have prognostic value?

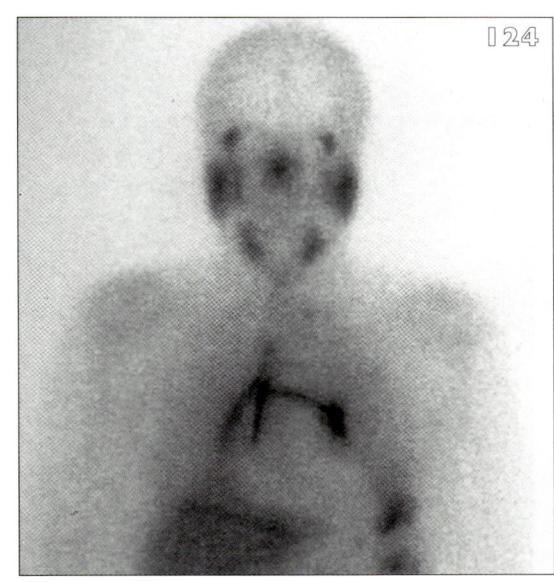

125 This collecting jar (**125**) is full of sputum. The patient, a 64-year-old man, filled it to 2 l in 2 days.
i. What is his phenomenon called?
ii. With what malignant lung disease is it associated?

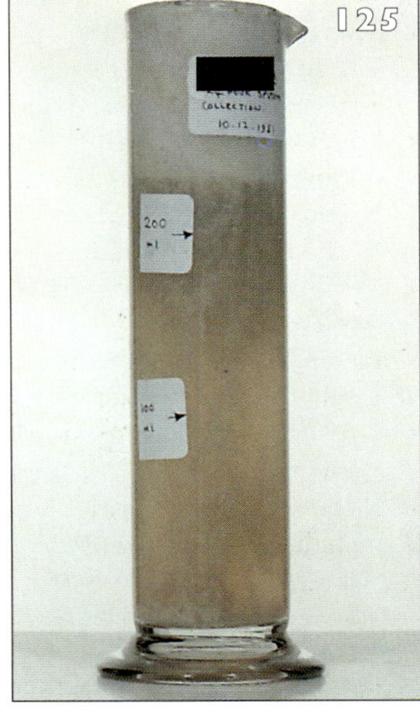

126 i. What are the main types of asbestos fibres?
ii. What are the risks to health from asbestos in homes and public buildings?

124 i. Physiological uptake occurs in the liver, bowel and breast with some uptake in the eyes and nose. It is taken up non-specifically in infections, inflammatory conditions and malignancy. Most scans are reported subjectively. In this patient there is increased uptake in the parotid and submandibular glands, lacrimal glands, hilar and mediastinal lymph nodes as well as the lungs. The parotid, lacrimal and hilar node uptake has been described as the 'panda–lambda' appearance, a phenomenon occurring in about 10% of sarcoid patients. This is highly specific and may obviate the need for histological confirmation in the presence of an elevated serum ACE in some patients. Pulmonary uptake can occur in most interstitial lung diseases. About 20% of patients with stage I disease have increased lung uptake despite clear lungfields on chest radiography.
ii. It cannot be recommended for routine use. It is useful for detecting sarcoidosis in selected patients such as a cardiomyopathy of unknown cause and to reassess patients with long-standing active disease.
iii. There are no studies that show conclusively that increased gallium uptake in the lungs correlates with prognosis.

125 i. The fluid is either saliva or sputum. The quantity is hugely excessive and sputum production at this rate is termed bronchorrhoea. Patients occasionally expectorate their saliva, complaining of excessive oral secretions, but sputum is more turbid and viscid and easy to distinguish from saliva.
ii. Alveolar cell carcinomas can cause bronchorrhoea due to the excessive mucous gland formation along the alveolar surfaces. It is untreatable with no response to cytotoxic chemotherapy, steroids or atropine. The chest radiograph will show a diffuse reticular distribution of disease, often extensive in one lung, and becoming bilateral quite commonly late in the disease.

126 i. The two main types are serpentine fibres such as chrysotile (White asbestos) and amphiboles (straight fibres) such as crocidolite (Blue asbestos)and amosite (Brown asbestos). Amphiboles are more capable of penetrating the lung periphery, whereas chrysotile fibres can be more readily removed from the lung by the mucociliary escalator. All fibre types are fibrogenic; however, amphiboles – particularly crocidolite – are more potent in terms of the development of mesothelioma. Most workers with asbestos have probably been exposed to a range of fibre types.
ii. Where asbestos has been used as an insulator around pipes and in walls and ceilings the greatest risk occurs when it is being removed, in which case workers must use respirators and protective clothing. At other times, where the surface of walls is not intact, there is a risk of asbestos dust being shed and subsequently inhaled. Where the surfaces are intact the risk of development of disease is thought to be negligible.

127 A patient with disseminated adenocarcinoma develops pain in the rib cage, left shoulder and right thigh. The pain is not controlled on eight paracetamol and codeine tablets a day. What steps would you take to control the pain and improve quality of life?

128 These bronchoscopic views (**128a, 128b**) are of the left main bronchus in a patient with inoperable lung cancer with recent increase in breathlessness.
i. What therapeutic strategy is appropriate?
ii. What has, in fact, been done?

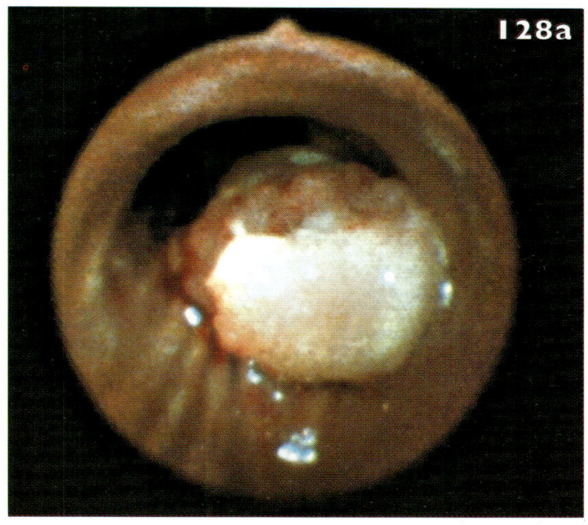

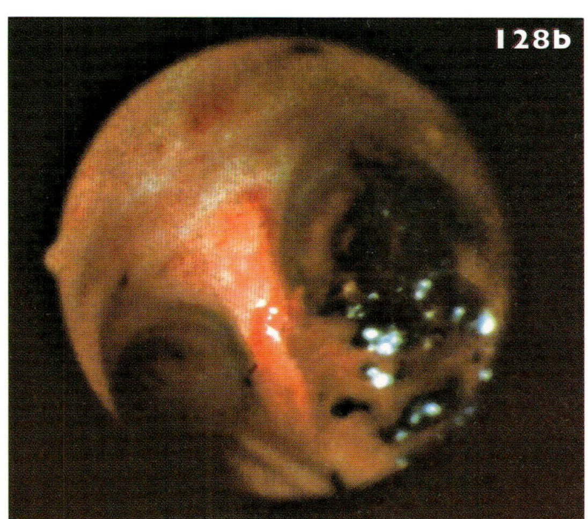

127 The pain is almost certainly due to bone metastases. If there is doubt, perform a bone scan (**127**). Bone pain is best initially treated with analgesics, such as paracetamol and codeine, together with a non-steroidal anti-inflammatory drug. The latter should be given as a slow-release preparation, i.e. b.d. or nocté.

If this is not adequate, short-term relief can be obtained by adding a corticosteroid. It is better to change the analgesics to a morphine preparation – ideally morphine sulphate continuos (MST) at 30–60 mg b.d. The non-steroidal drug should be continued. The patient should be warned about drowsiness for the first 2–3 days and of more sedation each time the dose of MST is increased. Breakthrough pain should be controlled by rapid-acting morphine (10 mg) tablets, which should be taken whenever necessary. An anti-nausea preparation should be routinely prescribed with the introduction of morphine, e.g. metoclopramide 10 mg q.d.s. or cyclizine

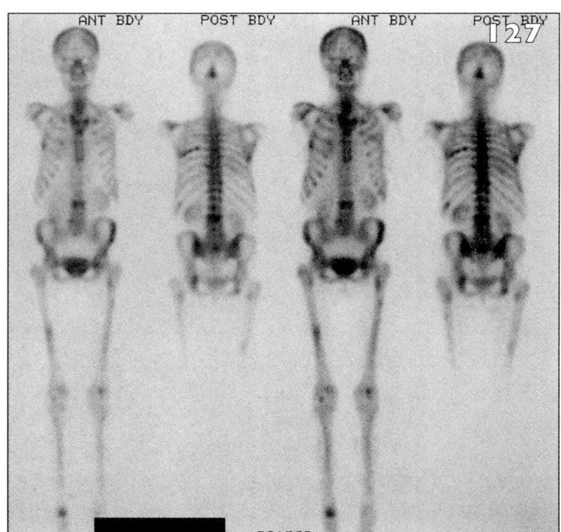

50 mg t.d.s. Also, an aperient is essential, either lactulose, 20–30 ml b.d. or co-danthrusate, 10–20 ml nocté. Do not be concerned about increasing the morphine b.d. dosage as control of pain is essential. Aperients may also have to be increased. Further medication that may be helpful is a tricyclic anti-depressant such as amitriptyline given at night. Very occasionally, nerve blocks or selective cordotomy can be effective for resistant, locally produced pain, although this is an unusual requirement with modern analgesia.

128 i. The tumour is in an intramural location in a major airway and there is no extrinsic compression. Therefore YAG laser resection is appropriate. The procedure is performed under general anaesthesia using a rigid bronchoscope through which the patient is ventilated and instruments are passed. A flexible glass fibre coated with protective cladding delivers the laser beam onto the tumour surface. As shown, an aiming beam, itself a helium–neon laser with no thermal properties, is used to show the point where the invisible YAG laser beam is being directed. The beam is fired into the tumour parallel to the bronchial wall to avoid direct penetration of the wall. The normal side of the bronchial tree must be kept free of secretions and blood to optimize oxygen delivery.

ii. This patient has received laser therapy with refashioning of the patent airway, as in **128b** which shows the procedure in progress with the laser fibre visible in the foreground.

129 The patient whose hand radiographs are depicted in **129** suffers from difficulty swallowing, arthralgias and a waxy appearance of her skin on her face and distal extremities.
i. What disorder accounts for these abnormalities?
ii. What are the two general types of pulmonary disease associated with this disorder?

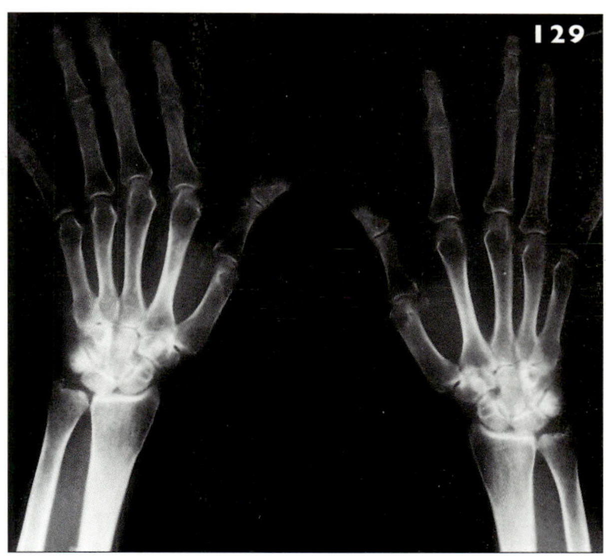

130 **i.** What procedure (**130a, 130b**) is this patient undergoing?
ii. What side effects may result from this treatment?

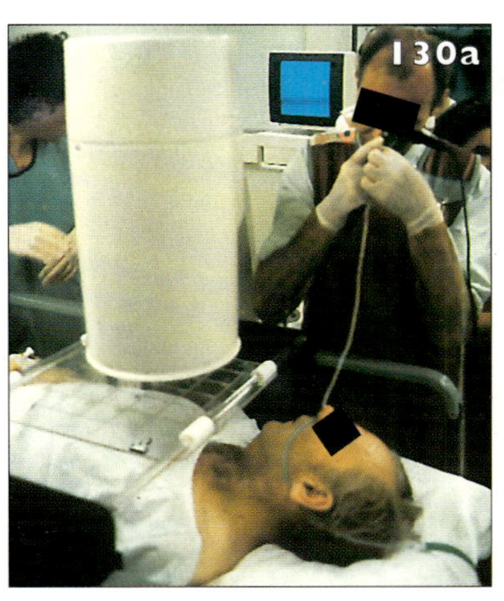

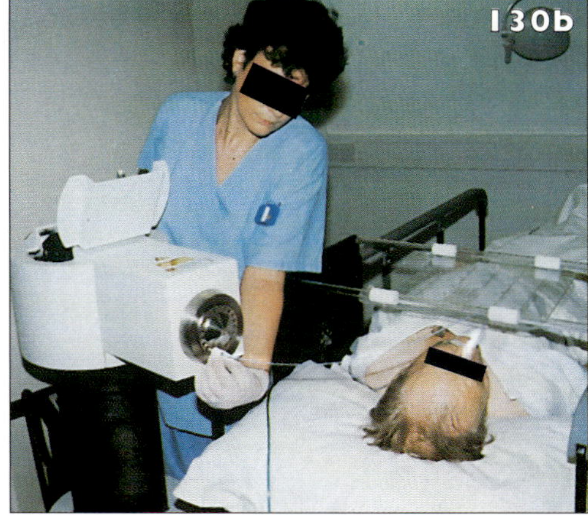

131 **i.** What are the most common infections following lung transplantation?
ii. What are the non-infective causes of lung damage following transplantation?

129 i. Progressive systemic sclerosis (or scleroderma) is a connective tissue disease in which progressive fibrosis and collagen replacement affects multiple organs, including the skin, oesophagus, joints and lung. The hand radiographs depict acro-osteolysis or erosion of the distal phalanges. Pulmonary symptoms include dyspnoea and cough.

ii. The most common pulmonary manifestation of systemic sclerosis is fibrosing alveolitis, the pattern of which is indistinguishable from idiopathic pulmonary fibrosis (CFA). A second, less common pulmonary manifestation is pulmonary hypertension. The severity of the pulmonary hypertension of progressive systemic sclerosis is not predicted by the degree of restrictive interstitial disease.

130 i. Endobronchial brachytherapy. Its role is primarily palliative for breathlessness but also for cough and haemoptysis. It is indicated for endobronchial tumour with a mural and or endobronchial component, preferably without extrinsic compression. Occasionally it may be used with curative intent in patients with small endobronchial tumours. It allows radiotherapy to be positioned and given directly to the tumour. Its effects take 10–14 days to become apparent and it is therefore of no use for acute relief of symptoms due to airway obstruction. However, it may be used as combined therapy with laser resection, stenting or external beam radiotherapy. The proximal and distal ends of the tumour are marked using the flexible bronchoscope and fluoroscopy. A catheter is then passed into the bronchus affected by tumour and the bronchoscope removed. Radioactive material, usually iridium (^{192}Ir) is then loaded into the distal end of a catheter using the Microselectron afterloading device as depicted. High-dose rate (HDR) brachytherapy is now the most common form of brachytherapy and 10–15 Gy is delivered over 10–20 min, with the maximum diameter of effect being 1 cm.

ii. The procedure is performed under local anaesthetic with intravenous sedation and is generally well tolerated.

131 i. The most common infections are:
- Bacterial: *P. aeruginosa*, *Str. pneumoniae*, *H. influenzae*, *Staph. aureus*, *B. cepacia*.
- Fungal: *A. fumigatus* and *C. albicans*.
- Viral: Cytomegalovirus.
- Other: *P. carinii*, *T. gondii*.

ii. The non-infective causes causing lung damage following transplantation are:
- Acute rejection, which occurs in nearly every patient in the first few months following transplantation.
- Obliterative bronchiolitis occurs in 40% of patients as a late complication of transplantation, probably due to previous lung injury which includes infection and rejection. It responds poorly to treatment and is the major cause of late mortality.
- Lymphoproliferative disorders due to T- or B-cell types. B-cells are usually associated with the Epstein–Barr virus.

132 This patient complained of dependent oedema, abdominal discomfort and chronic fatigue.
i. Describe the abnormality present in the radiograph (**132**).
ii. What is the likely aetiology?
iii. What are the pathological processes and what are the physiological consequences?
iv. What form of treatment is required?

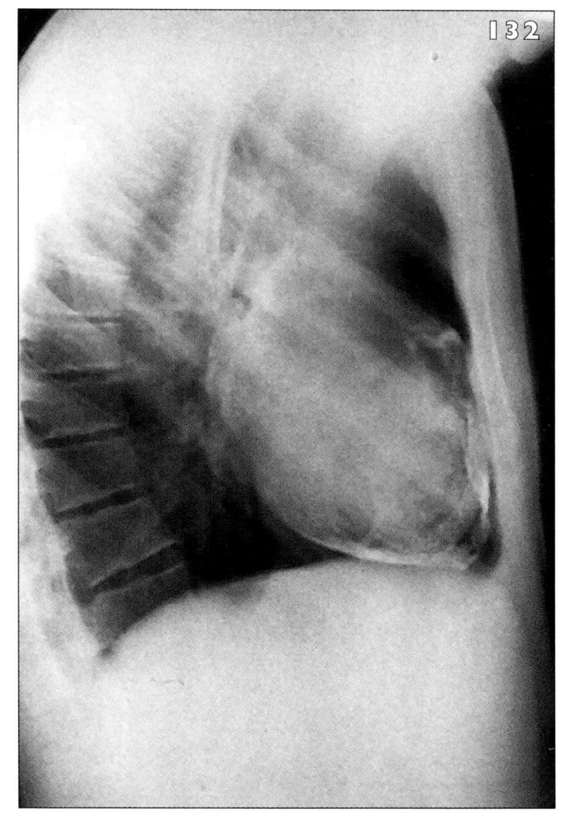

133 i. What is the mechanism of action of CPAP (**133**) in obstructive sleep apnoea?
ii. What are the potential side effects of nasal CPAP?
iii. How compliant are OSA patients who are prescribed CPAP?

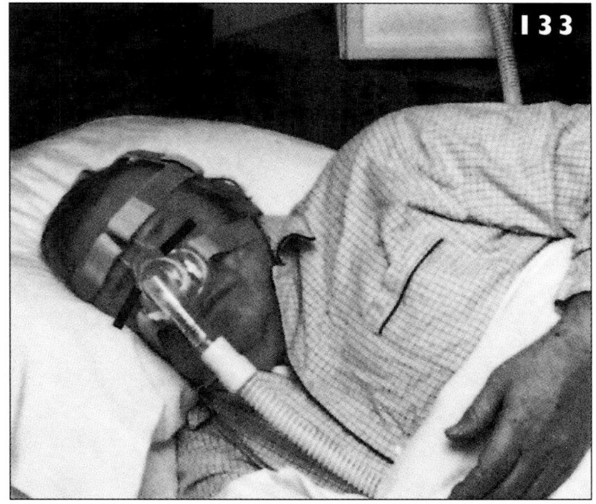

132 i. Pericardial calcification.
ii. Tuberculous pericarditis is the most likely aetiology, but calcification can occur following suppurative bacterial disease.
iii. The pericardial sac in this condition is obliterated by adhesions. The parietal pericardium is grossly thickened, fibrotic and calcified and the visceral pericardium is also rigid and fibrosed. There is consequently impaired diastolic filling as the heart cannot expand and venous inflow is further reduced by fibrous cuffing of the great veins as they enter the right atrium. Cardiac output is reduced and venous pressure chronically elevated causing hepatic engorgement, high jugular venous pressure and leg oedema. Residual foci of active TB are very rare.
iv. Pericardiectomy is required. This can be very difficult because of dense fibrosis and pericardial adhesions. It is usually necessary to either excise the visceral pericardium or to create multiple relieving incisions in order to adequately free the trapped myocardium and this increases the risk of haemorrhage or myocardial damage. Cardiac function can be very poor in the immediate postoperative period so that inotropic support is required and it may take many months to gain maximum benefit from the procedure. A pericardial specimen should be sent for culture and histology.

133 i. CPAP acts as a pneumatic splint. It increases the intraluminal pressure within the upper airway and thus counteracts transmural forces which favour airway closure. The typical site of obstruction in patients with OSA is between the nasopharynx and the larynx. This region is narrowed during sleep due to reduction in muscle tone, and OSA patients on average have a smaller diameter of pharyngeal lumen.
ii. Poorly fitting masks result in air leakage. This not only reduces the applied airway pressure, but also can cause conjunctivitis if the air leak is directed towards the eye. A poorly fitting mask can also bruise or cause ulceration of the bridge of the nose. These problems can be avoided by selecting and properly fitting the appropriate mask type and size. Most patients initially experience nasal congestion but this complaint frequently diminishes with continued use. Intranasal vasoconstrictors, anticholinergics or steroids have been used in this setting. Humidification of air within the CPAP system can also help if these measures are ineffective.
iii. Compliance rates vary from 45 to 80%. Many studies show average hours used to be less than 5 per night. There are no consistent clinical predictors of compliance, although one study suggested that patients who complain of side effects were those found to be less compliant. Follow-up and support by physicians and personalizing the type of CPAP device and mask may be important in improving patient compliance.

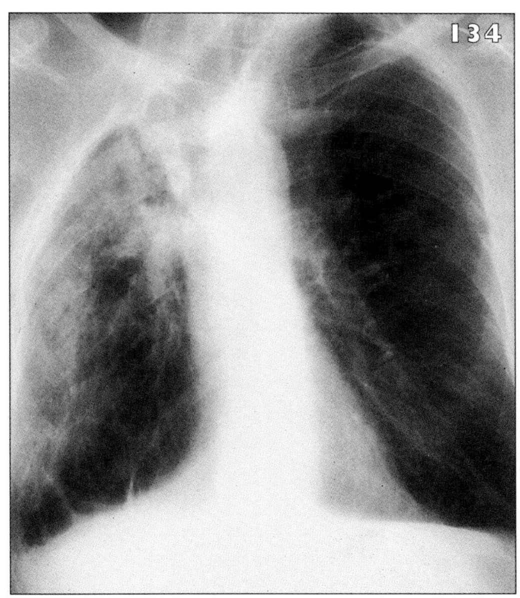

134 Shown is a chest radiograph (**134**) of a 70-year-old man with a 3-month history of cough, low-grade fever, weight loss and pulmonary infiltrates. As a young man, he had been successfully treated for pulmonary tuberculosis by thoracoplasty and right upper lobe resection. Multiple sputum specimens over the past 2 months were negative for tuberculosis by AFB stain. Mycobacterial, fungal and routine sputum cultures grew only mixed oral flora. Three 14-day courses of either erythromycin or ampicillin resulted in transient improvement that was followed by prompt recurrence of the symptoms. Bronchoalveolar lavage (BAL) cytology and transbronchial biopsies showed chronic inflammatory changes without evidence of neoplasm, granulomas or eosinophils. All BAL stains and cultures were negative, with the exception that quantitative bacterial cultures grew 500 cfu/ml of *Moraxella catarrhalis*. What is the most likely diagnosis and why?

135 i. How does a pulse oximeter work?
ii. The accuracy of most pulse oximeters decreases below what percent saturation?
iii. What factors affect the accuracy of pulse oximetry?

134 This patient has the chronic pneumonia syndrome, i.e. chronic symptoms of respiratory infection associated with radiographic abnormalities. The chronic and insidious nature of this syndrome suggests a variety of subacute, infectious processes including mycobacterial, fungal and parasitic diseases. Unusual bacterial infections (actinomycosis and nocardiosis) should also be considered, as should eosinophilic pneumonia (note the peripheral appearance of the infiltrate). Although less common, non-infectious lung diseases (e.g. neoplasms, connective tissue disease) can also present in this manner. Common bacterial respiratory pathogens rarely cause chronic pneumonia and usually do so only in patients with underlying diabetes, immunodeficiency or structural lung disease. Usual quantitative culture criteria for the diagnosis of bacterial pneumonia may not be applicable, and a prolonged course of antibiotic therapy appears necessary. Given the broad spectrum of potential causes for the chronic pneumonia syndrome, a comprehensive evaluation is warranted. In the absence of a relevant exposure history or systemic manifestations of an underlying disease, invasive diagnostic procedures may be necessary.

135 i. A pulse oximeter is a spectrophotometer which measures the absorption of light at two wavelengths; one in the infrared range at a wavelength of 940 nm (absorbed by oxyhaemoglobin) and the other at a wavelength of 660 nm (absorbed by reduced haemoglobin). The absorption at these two wavelengths is compared and the percentages of oxygenated and reduced haemoglobin calculated. The pulse oximeter compares absorption measured during systole and diastole and uses the difference to reflect only the absorption of arterial blood, thereby limiting errors induced by absorbance in venous blood and other tissues.
ii. The accuracy of most oximeters decreases below 75% saturation. Above this level, the accuracy is approximately 4%.
iii. Standard pulse oximeters are unable to distinguish dyshaemoglobins, most notably carboxyhaemoglobin and methaemoglobin, from oxyhaemoglobin. In smoke inhalation pulse oximetry reflects absorption by both oxyhaemoglobin and carboxyhaemoglobin, and thus may overestimate the true oxygenation status. Any factor which affects assessment of the arterial pulse (e.g., motion, low perfusion states) may distort the reading. Specific light sources, such as fluorescent or infrared lamps, can cause erroneous signals if the oximeter probe is not shielded. Dark skin pigmentation and darker coloured nail polishes can also interfere with light transmission, thereby lowering oximeter readings.

136 i. What is meant by a 'steady-state' exercise test?
ii. What is the additional information it can produce?

137 i. Shown in **137a** is a photomicrograph of normal human alveolar macrophages obtained by bronchoalveolar lavage and incubated *in vitro*. **137b** shows the same cell preparation after it has been incubated with interferon-gamma.
i. What are the primary functions of the alveolar macrophage?
ii. What are the roles of alveolar macrophage secretory products.

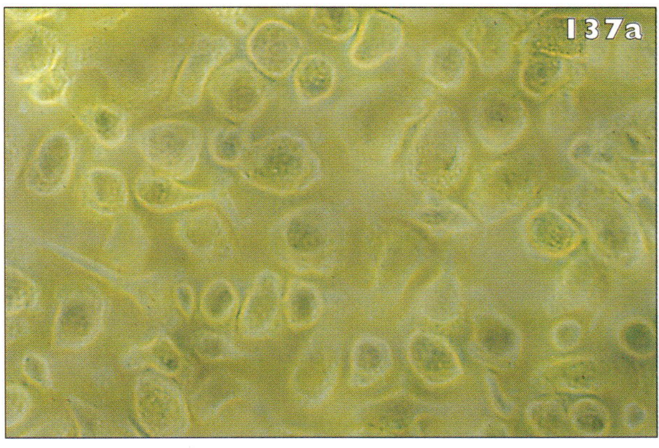

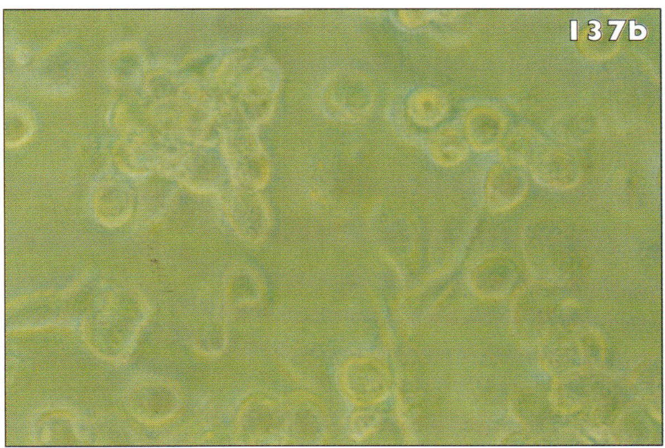

136 i. Steady-state exercise testing is usually performed at a work rate up to 50% of the maximum achieved by the subject during an earlier progressive exercise test, as shown in **136**. It allows the heart rate, minute ventilation and oxygen uptake to plateau after 3–4 minutes of exercise at a constant workload and it is usual for the test to be performed for 6 minutes.

ii. It is performed to measure heart rate, ventilation, mixed expired gases and arterial blood and to use this to calculate cardiac output, dead space, dead space:tidal volume ratio, the percentage of shunt through the lungs and the alveolar arterial oxygen gradient. These tests are usually only carried out in specialized laboratories if it is thought clinically useful to determine these parameters.

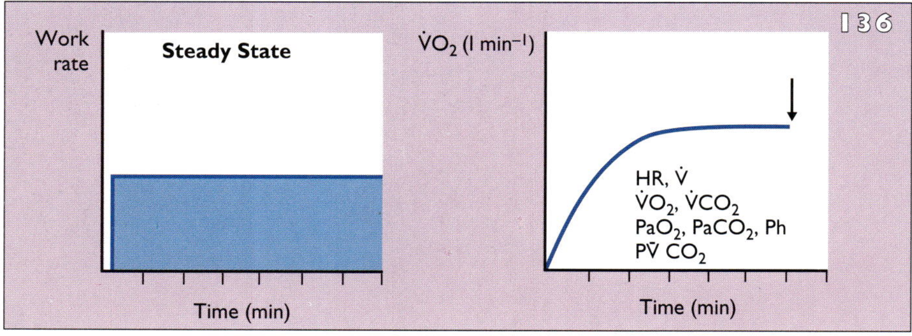

137 i. Alveolar macrophages are the resident phagocytic cells in the lung. They serve as scavengers of inhaled particulate material and senescent cells and are the sentinels against invasion of the lung by infectious agents.

ii. Non-specific scavenger receptors permit the alveolar macrophage to bind and ingest inert substances without initiating an inflammatory response. In contrast, the ingestion of infectious pathogens typically stimulates a brisk response that results in macrophage activation and inflammatory cell recruitment. These events are regulated by networks of secretory products, primarily cytokines. Interferon-gamma, produced by lymphocytes, is a potent macrophage-activating factor. The alveolar macrophage can also be activated by autocrine cytokines, including TNF, IL-1, and GM-CSF. These mediators promote morphological changes such as the spreading and clumping seen in **137b**. Metabolic changes include stimulation of the oxidative burst pathway, up-regulation of inflammatory cytokine production and increased expression of cell-surface receptors mediating adhesion, phagocytosis and antigen presentation. Other macrophage-derived cytokines, such as IL-10 and TGF, provide an autocrine negative feedback mechanism by down-regulating many of these macrophage functions. Macrophage-derived chemotactic factors, including leukotriene B4 and the IL-8 chemokine family, recruit neutrophils to the site of infection, while other products attract monocytes and lymphocytes. Additional interactions between macrophage-derived cytokines and epithelial cells, endothelial cells, fibroblasts and lymphocyte subpopulations further alter the inflammatory response.

138 Shown is the chest radiograph (138) of a 56-year-old woman from south-east Asia with chronic cough, malaise and weight loss. Multiple sputum specimens submitted for mycobacterial and fungal culture have yielded negative results.
i. What are the radiographic findings?
ii. What is the most likely diagnosis and how can this be established?
iii. What is the appropriate treatment?

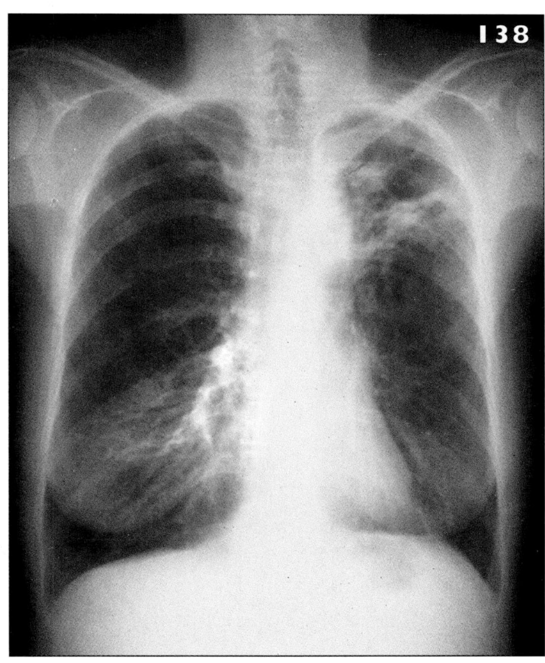

139 The chest radiograph in **139** is of a patient with cystic fibrosis (CF).
i. What does it show?
ii. Why is a spontaneous pneumothorax in CF different?
iii. What is the optimum medical management?
iv. What is the optimum surgical management?

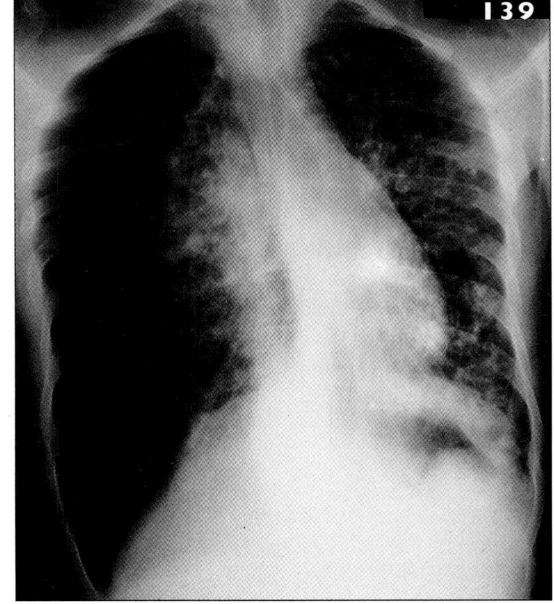

138 i. There is a cavitating infiltrate in the apical segment of the left upper lobe.
ii. Melioidosis is an important cause of respiratory infection in tropical regions, especially south-east Asia. It is caused by the Gram-negative bacterial pathogen, *P. pseudomallei*, yet it is acquired by cutaneous inoculation with haematogenous spread to the lungs. Melioidosis may present acutely, with evidence of cellulitis at the inoculation site, prominent systemic and respiratory symptoms, and diffuse pulmonary infiltrates. A more insidious or chronic form of the disease may develop long after an infected patient leaves the endemic area. The presentation of chronic melioidosis is characterized by indolent wasting symptoms, cough and apical infiltrates which may become fibrotic or cavitating – features indistinguishable from pulmonary tuberculosis. The diagnosis of melioidosis should be considered whenever a compatible syndrome develops in a patient who has been in an endemic area. The organism can readily be cultured from respiratory secretions or other sites, and infection can be confirmed by serologic testing.
iii. *P. pseudomallei* is sensitive to a variety of antimicrobial agents, but resistance is variable and antibiotic selection should be based on *in vitro* sensitivity testing. For acute disease, combination intravenous therapy including an aminoglycoside is recommended for 1 month followed by several months of oral treatment. For chronic disease, a 3- to 6-month course of an oral agent such as trimethoprim/sulphamethoxazole may be used.

139 i. A large right tension pneumothorax. The incidence of pneumothorax increases with disease severity and may be associated with a poor prognosis. It occurs due to rupture of subpleural blebs through the visceral pleura, usually in the upper lobes. The incidence of pneumothorax is higher in patients with widespread pre-existing lung disease.
ii. A pneumothorax in CF is different from that occurring in other patients due to its association with large amounts of purulent secretions. This can make physiotherapy difficult and lung re-expansion very slow. In addition, CF patients who get pneumothoraces usually have severe disease and with a pneumothorax can become extremely sick.

Patients with pneumothoraces need prompt medical treatment. At the time of the pneumothorax they should be commenced on intravenous antibiotics. If large it should be drained immediately. If the patient is breathless a small pneumothorax requires intercostal drainage under radiological control. An intubated pneumothorax makes physiotherapy easier. A small pneumothorax in an asymptomatic patient may be aspirated or observed for 2–3 days.
iii. If a pneumothorax fails to resolve with maximal medical management within a week then prompt surgical intervention should be considered.
With the advent of organ transplantation extensive pleurodesis or pleurectomy are not appropriate. The best surgical option is video-assisted stapling of the apical subpleural bleb under direct vision.

140 i. What operation has this patient undergone (140)?
ii. How should the procedure be monitored postoperatively?

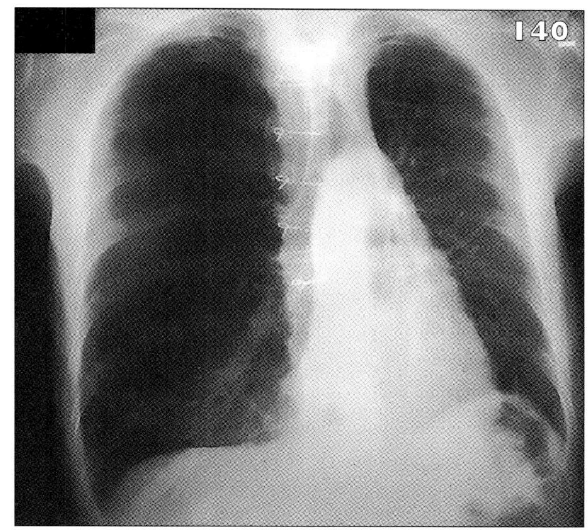

141 These high-resolution chest CTs (141a, 141b) are from a 37-year-old man who presented with a spontaneous pneumothorax.
i. What diagnosis does the CT suggest?
ii. What is the typical clinical presentation of this disease?
iii. What abnormalities are seen on histopathological examination?

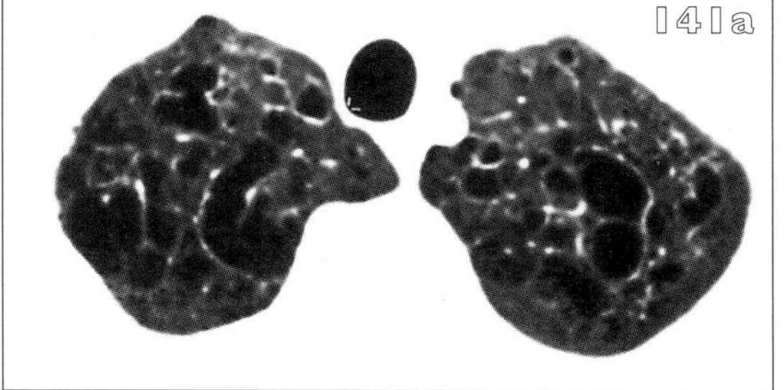

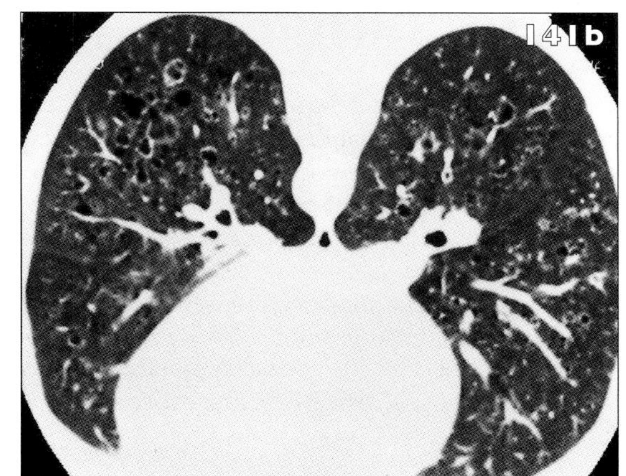

140 i. Left single lung transplant for COPD (still evident in the right lung).
ii. Patients perform a vital role in monitoring for the complications of lung transplantation which include infection related to immunposuppression, graft rejection and anastomotic complications. Cough, breathlessness, fever and falling peak flow measurements may herald any of these complications and should be investigated promptly. In addition, regular transbronchial lung biopsies are performed in some centres to monitor for the development of graft rejection. Chest radiographs may not show evidence of early graft rejection, particularly after 3 months. Rejection may be hyperacute, acute or chronic and results from host T-cell activation due to MHC molecule cell surface differences between host and donor. Acute rejection occurs up to 12 months and most patients have at least two episodes. Histology ranges from infrequent perivascular infiltrates of inflammatory cells to diffuse perivascular, interstitial and airspace infiltrates with an ARDS-like picture. Biopsies and lavage are also screened for infection which may coexist. Chronic rejection usually arises at 8–12 months with variable symptoms and progressive airflow obstruction. It occurs in 40% of cases remains a significant cause of late mortality. Histologically it manifests as bronchiolitis obliterans.

Bronchoscopy is also useful for surveillance of the anastomosis site for complications such as bronchial strictures which may require stent placement or surgery, or dehiscence which requires reoperation.

141 i. Eosinophilic granuloma. The major findings on chest CT are irregular, cystic structures of variable size, most being 3–5 cm in diameter (**141a**), suggestive of eosinophilic granuloma. The chest radiograph in this disorder is characterized by diffusely increased interstitial markings. A nodular or reticular nodular infiltrate is present, sometimes accompanied by cystic lesions (**141b**). Most commonly the infiltrate is found in the lung periphery and in the upper lobes. Volume loss is characteristically absent on both the chest radiograph and the CT.
ii. Primary pulmonary histiocytosis X or eosinophilic granuloma of the lung can present at any age, but is most frequently seen in the third and fourth decades of life. Patients complain of cough and exertional dyspnoea, but may be asymptomatic. Spontaneous pneumothorax is a classical association. Progressive decline in lung function and the occurrence of multiple pneumothoraces implies a poor long-term prognosis. Pleurodesis may be of use in these patients. Immunosuppressive treatment is of unproven value. The eosinophilic granulomata can also occur in the pituitary gland causing diabetes insipidus and may cause asymptomatic bone cysts, detected on a radiological skeletal survey.
iii. The classical pathological findings are discrete parenchymal nodules composed of fibrous tissue, eosinophils and 'histiocytosis X' cells which resemble Langerhans cells of the skin. These histiocytosis cells are characterized by intracytoplasmic X bodies which may be visualized by electron microscopy.

142 This 45-year-old, non-smoking man produced the flow–volume curve in **142**.

i. Is it of normal or abnormal shape?

ii. What is point A? How is it usually measured?

iii. Why does the expiratory curve decrease progressively in flow as the residual volume is approached?

iv. Why is the inspiratory curve semi-circular in shape and dissimilar to the expiratory curve?

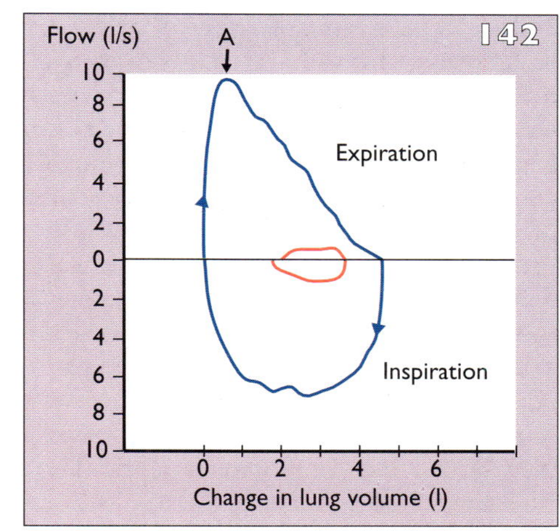

143 This patient (**143**) had polio 30 years ago and was clinically stable until recently when he developed fatigue, joint pains, muscle weakness, swallowing difficulties and dyspnoea.

i. What disorder does this patient have and what are the underlying factors responsible for his breathing abnormality?

ii. How is sleep affected in this disorder?

iii. How is this disorder managed?

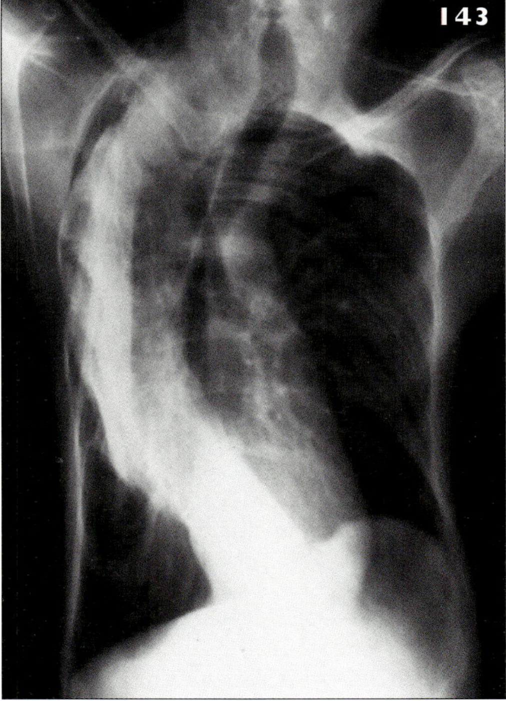

142 i. This is a normal-shaped curve.

ii. The expiratory limb is triangular in shape. Following a full inspiration, the lung's recoil pressure is maximal, as is pleural pressure, because the thoracic muscles are stretched to provide maximal expiratory force. The onset of expiratory flow is explosive and reaches its peak rate within 0.01 s, i.e. point A. This is the peak expiratory flow rate and is usually measured with a peak flow meter.

iii. The expiratory curve decreases its flow gradually as the lung volume drops from total lung capacity to residual volume. This graded decline reflects the gradual drop in the lung's elastic recoil as the lung gets smaller; also, muscular force on the lung (pleural pressure) slowly decreases as the thoracic cage changes position during expiration and the respiratory muscles shorten.

iv. Inspiration does not reach an instant maximal flow in contrast to expiration. As the respiratory muscles contract, the power increases progressively from the start of inspiration to achieve a maximal flow. This takes a relatively long time and maximal inspiratory flow is only achieved by the mid-point of the inspiratory vital capacity; it then slows again as the maximum inspired volume is reached (total lung capacity; TLC). This results in the semi-circular appearance of the inspiratory flow–volume curve.

143 i. This patient has the post-polio syndrome which usually occurs two to three decades after the acute infection and recovery. These patients usually have kyphoscoliosis which causes restriction and can blunt the hypercapnic drive because of mechanical impairment. In addition, they may also have decreased respiratory drive as a result of damage to their medullary neurones and may also have respiratory muscle weakness. Patients who did not have respiratory involvement with the initial infection are unlikely to develop such weakness or kyphoscoliosis.

ii. In the early stages, respiration during sleep is more likely to be affected. Initially, short central apnoeas occur and as the condition progresses these become longer and more frequent. Sleep abnormalities include decreased sleep efficiency and increased arousal frequency. Eventually, awake respiration can be affected.

iii. Patients with predominantly central sleep apnoea should be managed with bi-level positive airway pressure during sleep which is delivered via a nasal mask. A 20 cmH$_2$O inspiratory pressure support can be achieved with this, with expiratory support of 5 cm H$_2$O delivering a defined number of breaths. This must be timed support, per minute rather than triggered by the patient's breathing. Some patients who have more severe disease which includes irregularities in awake breathing, will require ventilatory support both during sleep and wakefulness. Early ventilation systems included negative-pressure tank apparatus. Nasal positive pressure ventilation is now more commonly used.

144 This woman developed a rash (144) 1 month after completing cytotoxic chemotherapy for small-cell lung cancer. What is the rash? Why did she develop it? How would you treat it?

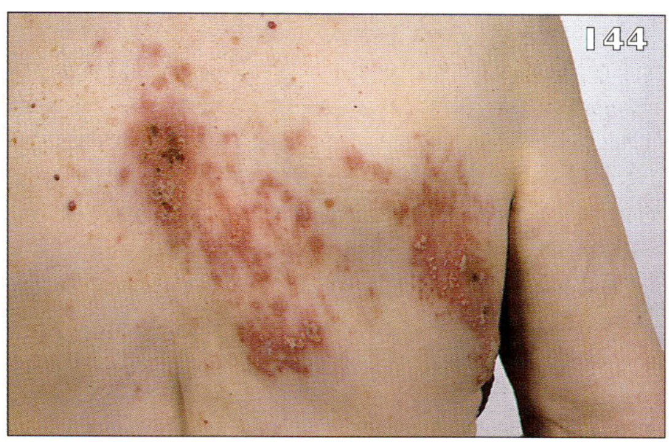

145 A 62-year-old woman is noted to have a low diffusing capacity during evaluation for dyspnoea.
i. What does the diffusing capacity measure?
ii. What physiological abnormalities result in a low diffusing capacity and what diagnoses might be associated with these abnormalities?
iii. What effect would anaemia have on the value?

146 This 68-year-old man had been unwell for 2 weeks, with a dry cough, dyspnoea and drenching sweats. What do the radiographs 146a and 146b show, what are the likely causes and how should the condition be managed?

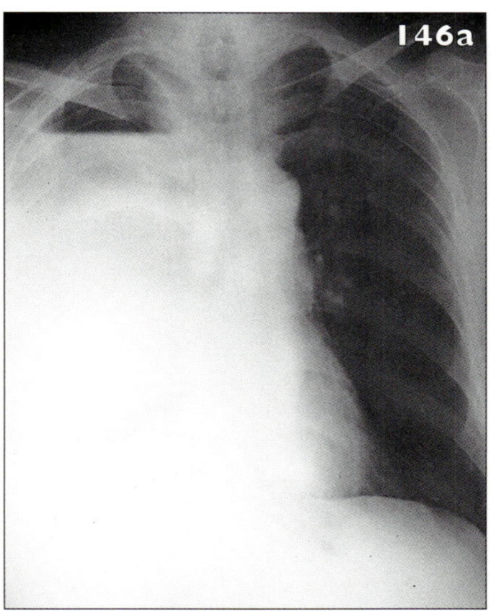

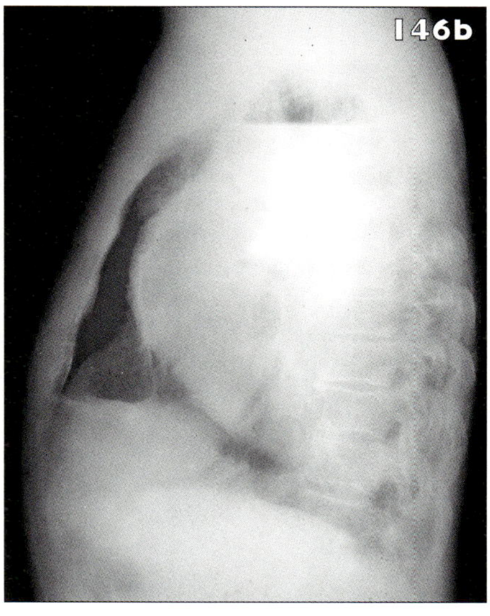

144 The rash is due to infection with herpes zoster, i.e. shingles. It occurs most commonly in immunosuppressed patients and is not uncommonly seen during or after a course of cytotoxic chemotherapy. The more widespread the underlying cancer, the greater the prospect of significant immunosuppression and hence the increased likelihood of developing shingles.

If the shingles is severe, and painful, treatment initially should be with i.v. acyclovir four to five times a day for 2 days and then orally for a further 3 days. Treatment is only likely to be effective if commenced within 48 h of symptoms commencing.

145 i. The diffusing capacity (DL_{CO}) measures the amount of carbon monoxide that transfers from a volume of inspired gas into the blood over a standard time – usually 10 s.
ii. The test is sensitive to reductions in diffusing surface (e.g. emphysema, lung resection, effusions, pneumothorax, atelectasis, bronchiolitis obliterans, fibrosis) and capillary blood volume (pulmonary emboli or other pulmonary vascular disease).
iii. A low haemoglobin may lead to an erroneous interpretation of the diffusing capacity as there is a reduced capacity of the blood in the alveolar capillaries to carry CO (and O_2) away. The correction of DL_{CO} for anaemia should be routine in all pulmonary function laboratories. The DL_{CO} falls by 7% for each 1 g/100 ml fall in haemoglobin.

146 Pleural empyema. This is usually a complication of an acute pneumonia – particularly pneumococcal – but may arise as a primary infection of the pleural space, in which case the organism is often an anaerobe producing 'stinking pus'. A tuberculous pleural effusion may also progress to an empyema, particularly if a cavity ruptures into the pleural space. A previous history of vomiting and aspiration is not uncommon and carcinoma of the bronchus is also a predisposing factor.

Empyemas tend to adhere to the chest wall, causing loculated collections of fluid. This differs from a simple pleural effusion and the lateral chest radiograph (**146b**) here confirms a large quantity of fluid adherent to the posterior aspect of the left thoracic cage.

Thorough pleural drainage with a wide-bore intercostal tube is imperative and should be done as soon as possible. Recent studies have shown that daily intrapleural installations of streptokinase break down adhesions and greatly improve drainage. Systemic antibiotics must also be given, usually for several weeks to clear the infection. Thorough lavage of the cavity, in order to remove infected fibrin and debris, also encourages resolution. In some cases, despite vigorous treatment, it may be necessary to perform a surgical decortication. This should be done, if possible, several weeks after antibiotic therapy is completed to remove a thick cortex of debris which has prevented adequate re-expansion of the lung.

147 The radiograph **147** is from a patient with CF.
i. What concomitant condition does it show?
ii. What is the optimum treatment?

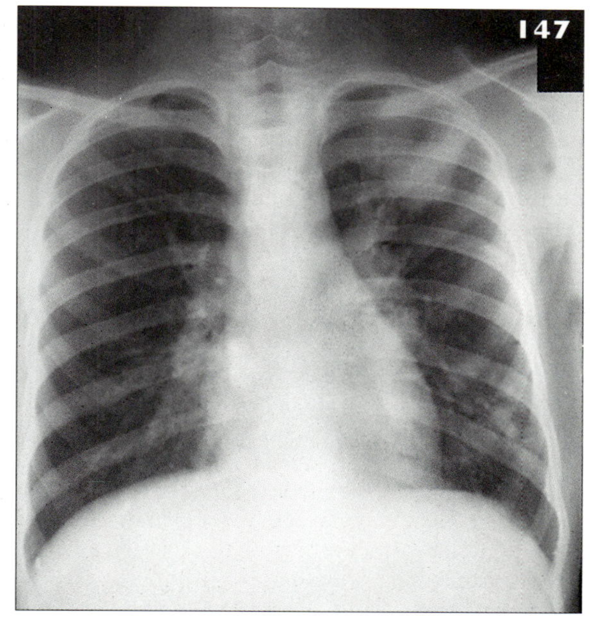

148 This nurse (**148**) is inserting a cleaning agent into an automated bronchoscope washer.
i. Which respiratory condition might she develop?
ii. Which other hospital professionals may develop this?
iii. Which infectious organisms may resist cleaning?

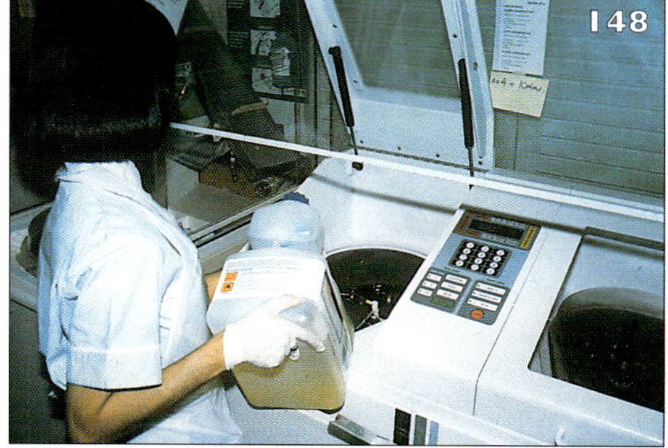

147 i. Allergic bronchopulmonary aspergillosis (ABPA). Changes due to CF are not particularly marked, but the rounded lesions and linear shadows in the left lower lobe are bronchiectatic airways. There is bronchial wall thickening in the upper lobe confluent with an area of consolidation. Although consolidation due to infection is possible, the airway damage and presence of CF make ABPA possible. Classically the shadowing in ABPA is particular and associated with proximal bronchiectasis. The role of *A. fumigatus* in the pathology of CF pulmonary disease is complex. The organism is commonly found in the sputum of 50% of patients and precipitins are associated with increased disease severity, but ABPA may not be present.
ii. The optimum treatment for a definite diagnosis of ABPA in CF is oral corticosteroids. These may need to be long term. A reduction in total IgE levels is the best monitor of a response to treatment.

Antifungal agents (itraconazole) have been used with some success but there are no published long-term controlled trials.

148 i. The cleaning agent is glutaraldehyde which can cause occupational asthma, hence the use of the fume cabinet and the enclosed washer. Glutaraldehyde is an airway sensitizer, and may also cause skin hypersensitivity and irritant effects on the eyes and throat. Onset of symptoms is usually after an interval of months to years from first exposure. Symptoms usually improve after returning home from work each day. If peak flow records are suggestive, specific bronchial provocation tests can be performed with glutaraldehyde to prove the diagnosis. In keeping with the airway-sensitizing effects, there may be a delayed reaction to the inhaled glutaraldehyde on bronchial provocation, although immediate reactions are also seen. Glutaraldehyde is also contained in radiographic film developer, and is used as a fixative in electron microscopy.
ii. Other hospital professionals who may come into contract with substances that cause occupational asthma include radiography technicians, mortuary workers and pathologists (formaldehyde), orthopaedic surgeons and nurses, and dentists (adhesives), those using and handling latex rubber gloves or chlorhexidine, and research workers exposed to laboratory animals.
iii. Glutaraldehyde is the most effective cold sterilizing agent for bronchoscopes. However, very occasional transmission of infection from bronchoscopes may occur with atypical mycobacteria, *Pseudomonas* spp., *Serratia marcescens* and *Bacillus* spp. A 10-min soak in glutaraldehyde should inactivate all viruses and bacteria, whereas 1 hour is recommended for mycobacteria.

149 Patient A has a large left pleural effusion and a single breath gas transfer factor (DL_{CO}) of 55% normal along with a transfer coefficient (K_{CO}) of 90% normal. Patient B with bullous emphysema has a DL_{CO} of 55%.
i. What is the K_{CO}? How is it measured?
ii. Why does the K_{CO} in Patient A correct to near normal?
iii. What is the K_{CO} likely to be in Patient B (i.e. high, normal or low) and why?

150 You are called to see an 81-year-old smoker who 24 hours after an elective cholecystectomy has developed respiratory distress, fever, a cough and a left lower lobe infiltrate on the chest radiograph.
i. What is the most likely causative organism?
He deteriorates and is admitted to intensive care for intubation and assisted ventilation. He responds well to initial treatment but 1 week later deteriorates and develops further bilateral shadowing while still on the ventilator.
ii. What is the most likely cause for this change?

151 These lung function tests (Table) are from a 42-year-old woman with progressive systemic sclerosis. Chest and cardiac examination were normal, as was the chest radiograph. What is the pathogenesis of the abnormality?

Test	Predicted	Range	Result	% predicted
FEV$_1$ (l)	2.10	1.79–2.42	2.10	100
FVC (l)	2.84	2.42–3.26	2.50	88
FEV$_1$ (%)	73	62–84	83	115
FRC (l)	3.00	2.55–3.45	2.42	81
TLC (l)	5.18	4.40–5.96	4.32	83
VC (l)	2.84	2.41–3.26	2.44	86
RV (l)	1.90	1.62–2.19	1.88	99
DL_{CO} (mmol/min/kPa)*	7.23	6.15–8.31	3.48	48
VA(l)	–	–	3.73	–
K_{CO} (mmol/min/kPa/l)**	1.65	1.40–1.90	0.93	56

*DL_{CO} = transfer factor. **K_{CO} = transfer coefficient in DL_{CO}/VA.

149 i. The K_{CO} is the single breath gas transfer factor (DL_{CO}) corrected by the alveolar volume (VA). The alveolar volume is measured by an inert gas technique – usually using helium – which is inspired together with the carbon monoxide. As the helium is inert, it will not escape from the lungs and the dilutional decrease measured on expiration will give the alveolar volume, that is, the volume of lung that saw the helium and, therefore, the carbon monoxide, i.e. it is the amount of volume that was available under the circumstances of this test for gas exchange. The DL_{CO} divided by the alveolar volume gives the transfer coefficient, which is the quality of gas exchange in those areas of the lungs that were available to the two gases.
ii. The K_{CO} in Patient A corrects to near normal as the alveolar volume will be essentially that of the non-affected lung, i.e. the right lung.
iii. Here, the K_{CO} is likely to be low. In a patient with emphysema, the DL_{CO} will be low because of poor ventilation and perfusion due to parenchymal damage. The lung volumes, however, will be normal or larger than normal and the alveolar volume will be normal or high. Correcting a low DL_{CO} by a normal or high alveolar volume will give a low K_{CO}. This low K_{CO} (often very low) is characteristic of emphysema.

150 i. Although this is a postoperative pneumonia the most likely causes are the bacteria which are normal commensals in the oropharynx, so *Strep. pneumoniae* and *H. influenzae* would be the most common causes of pneumonia occurring this soon after hospital admission. The antibiotic treatment therefore is as for any other community-acquired pneumonia. At his age, so-called atypical organisms such as mycoplasma, chlamydia, coxiella or legionella would be unlikely.
ii. This time, nosocomial (hospital-acquired) infection is the most likely cause of his lung shadowing although other non-infective causes of lung shadowing such as pulmonary oedema or pulmonary infarction would need to be considered. The most common cause of nosocomial pneumonias are Gram-negative enterobacteria, followed by staphylococci; in the intensive care setting, *P. aeruginosa* is perhaps the most common and most difficult to deal with. The treatment of choice would be with a combination of a third generation cephalosporin which has anti-pseudomonal cover, with or without an aminoglycoside.

151 Reduction of gas transfer is often the earliest abnormality seen on pulmonary function tests in these patients and may be due to pulmonary vascular disease or fibrosing alveolitis. The preservation of lung volumes here suggests pulmonary vascular disease. Small pulmonary arteries and arterioles become narrowed due to marked intimal thickening by myxomatous connective tissue. Sequelae are pulmonary hypertension, which may improve with nifedipine if detected early, and eventually cor pulmonale. Pulmonary vascular effects and fibrotic pulmonary disease can occur independently but often the two pathologies are combined.

152 This 72-year-old woman presented with a 3-month history of malaise, sweats, weight loss, cough and occasional haemoptysis. She developed a pneumonia which was treated with antibiotics but responded poorly and she remained unwell with a low-grade fever. She was mildly anaemic with an ESR of 120 mm in 1 hour and a C-reactive protein (CRP) of 92.

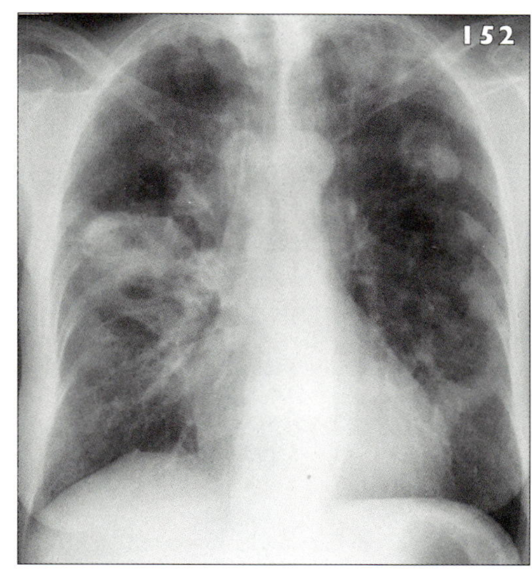

i. What does the radiograph (**152**) show and what is the differential diagnosis?
ii. How would you make the correct diagnosis?
iii. How would you treat the patient?

153 The peak flow chart shown in **102** was recorded by a patient with exertional breathlessness.
i. Is it consistent with asthma?
ii. How would you proceed?

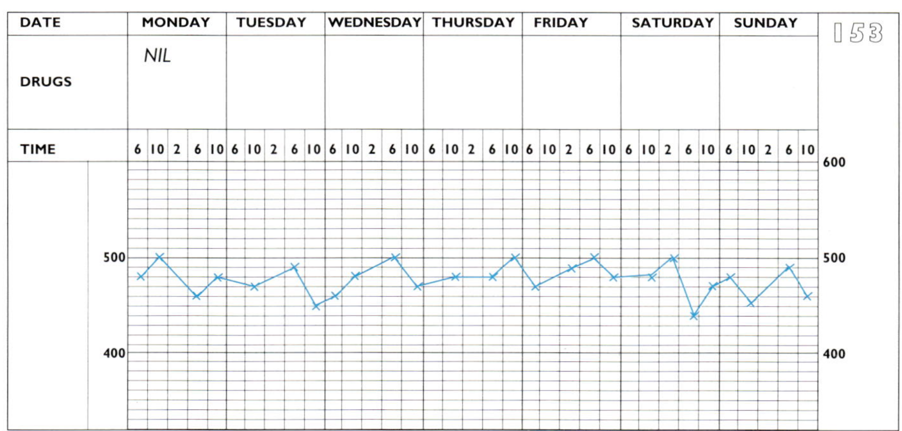

DATE	MONDAY	TUESDAY	WEDNESDAY	THURSDAY	FRIDAY	SATURDAY	SUNDAY	
DRUGS	NIL							153
TIME	6 10 2 6 10	6 10 2 6 10	6 10 2 6 10	6 10 2 6 10	6 10 2 6 10	6 10 2 6 10	6 10 2 6 10	

152 i. The chest radiograph shows multiple lesions of variable size throughout both lung fields and most have cavitated. The differential diagnosis includes staphylococcal pneumonia, lymphoma, TB, cavitating squamous cell carcinoma and a vasculitis – most likely Wegener's granulomatosis.

ii. This woman had Wegener's granulomatosis. The diagnosis was made by identifying c-ANCA (anti-cytoplasmic antibodies) in high titre in the peripheral blood. This is positive in more than 90% of cases and negative in classic polyarteritis nodosa and other vasculitidies. The titres of c-ANCA parallel disease activity and returned to normal when the disease is in remission. They can predict reactivation if a rise is detected in patients in remission.

iii. Untreated disease is fatal with a median survival of 5 months. The treatment of Wegener's granulomatosis, whether confined to the lung or more extensive with renal involvement, is with prednisolone and cyclophosphamide. In general, prednisolone is given at 1 mg/kg for 4 weeks and then slowly tailed down to a maintenance of 10 mg/day. Cyclophosphamide commences at 100–150 mg orally, and this is reduced by 25 mg every 2–3 months to 50 mg/day. Treatment is continued for 1 year after remission is achieved. Some 75% of patients achieve a complete remission and a further 15% a partial remission. Serial c-ANCA titres should be performed to predict relapse, which can occur in up to 50% of cases. The prognosis is better for Wegener's that is confined to the lungs.

153 i. No. The diagnosis of asthma is supported if peak flow variations of at least 20% occur between the highest and lowest readings, especially if the lowest readings occur repeatedly in the mornings. Although the chart shows variability it is within normal limits as peak flows in normal patients may vary up to 8%. This variability is due to circadian variation, with airway calibre being narrowest early in the mornings. The causes of this are thought to include diurnal rhythm of cortisol and catecholamine secretion and vagal tone, as well as reduced nocturnal mucociliary clearance.

ii. One non-supportive peak flow chart does not exclude asthma. The symptoms should be reviewed looking for cough, wheeze or breathlessness with diurnal variation. If still suspected, either repeating the PEFR record (stressing the need for measurements during symptomatic periods) or a 2-week trial of inhaled therapy may be performed. If the peak flow chart is undiagnostic a bronchial provocation test can be performed with increasing concentrations of inhaled methacoline. Bronchial hyperreactivity, if present, is strongly suggestive of asthma.

154 These chest radiographs (**154a**, **154b**) were obtained in an asymptomatic 65-year-old retired pipe fitter with a history of substantive exposure to asbestos.
i. What are the primary abnormalities on **154a** and **154b**?
ii. What is the differential diagnosis for these abnormalities?
iii. What is the significance of these findings?

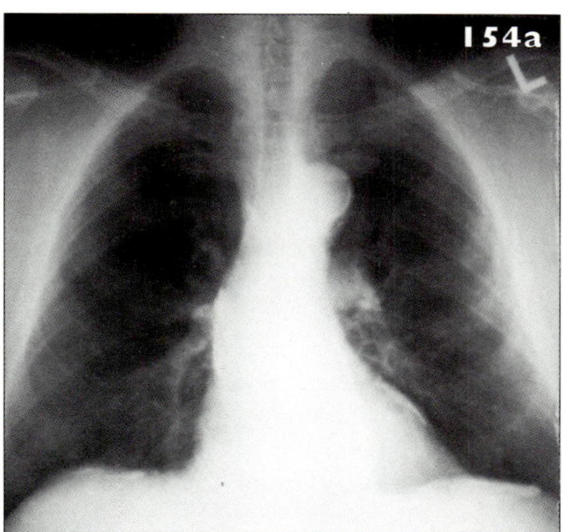
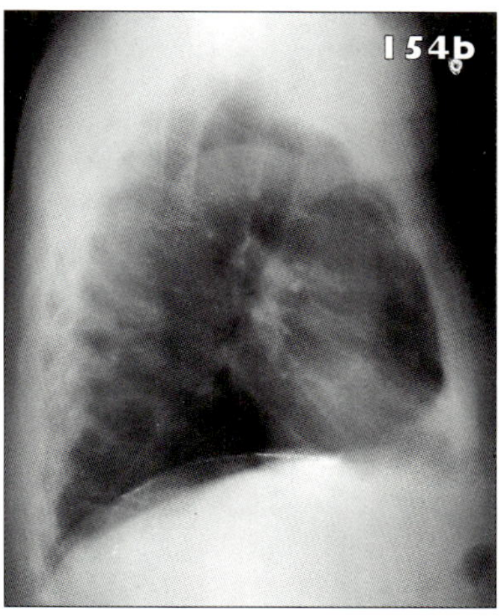

155 i. What is the impact of OSA on mortality?
ii. Name some illnesses associated with nocturnal death.
iii. What is thought to be the risk factor associated with these nocturnal deaths?

156 Shown (**156**) is a swollen right ankle and diffuse macular rash in a young female with CF.
i. What is the diagnosis?
ii. What is the medical treatment and prognosis?

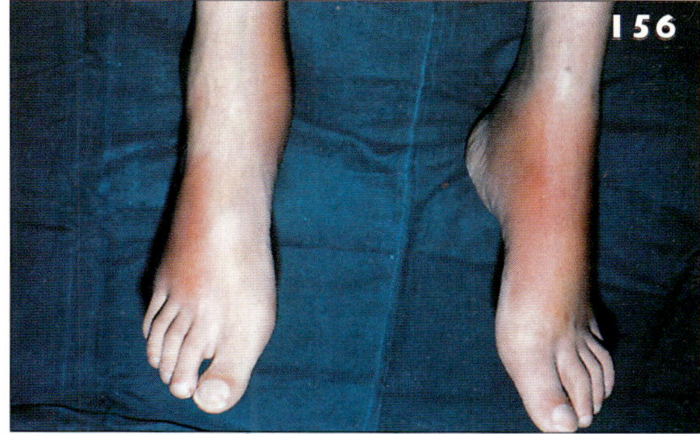

154 i. Bilateral calcified diaphragmatic plaques. Radiologically, uncalcified *en face* plaques appear as indistinct hazy opacities while plaques seen on edge appear as linear or oval pleural thickening. Calcified plaques can appear as irregular densities or dense linear opacifications along the diaphragm or chest wall.

ii. Extrapleural fat in more obese patients and serratus anterior shadows may be confused with uncalcified lateral chest wall plaques but are usually symmetrical bilaterally. A CT scan often resolves this uncertainty. Pleural calcification may develop following traumatic haemothorax, pleural tuberculosis and empyema, but is usually unilateral. Bilateral pleural calcification may occur in scleroderma and following exposure to mica and talc.

iii. Pleural plaques are the most common manifestation of asbestos exposure, eventually developing in 30–50% of exposed workers with a mean latency from first exposure to diagnosis of 20 years. In general, the extent of pleural involvement correlates with the intensity and duration of asbestos exposure. Plaques are bilateral, though not necessarily symmetric, and they are predominantly located on the mid-thoracic chest wall, adjacent to the ribs, in the paravertebral gutters, and over the central diaphragmatic tendon. Historically, pleural plaques have been considered to be a marker of asbestos exposure without any physiological effect. Recently, however, a statistically significant association between pleural plaques and reductions in forced vital capacity has been shown. The interpretation of these studies remains somewhat controversial, however, and isolated pleural plaques without coexistent parenchymal fibrosis likely have little, if any, clinically significant effects on lung function.

155 i. In a study of elderly women in nursing homes, those with a respiratory disturbance index of over 50 events per hour survived only 17% as long as those with an index of less than 30, and all those with an index over 50 died at night. However, it is still uncertain whether OSA is an independent risk factor over its common associations such as hypertension, obesity and increased body mass index.

ii. Asthma, coronary heart disease and the sudden infant death syndrome.

iii. The lack of autonomic nervous system control during rapid eye movement sleep may represent a risk period for health and may be a precipitating factor in nocturnal death.

156 i. This illustration shows a diffuse vasculitis involving the skin and synovium. Vasculitis of the skin may also be nodular or purpuric (without thrombocytopenia). It is associated with severe pulmonary disease and chronic *P. aeruginosa* infection. It has been attributed to the overspill into the systemic circulation of immune complexes resulting from the hyperimmune stimulation associated with chronic pulmonary disease.

ii. Medical treatment consists of short-term, high-dose oral steroids. This will usually produce complete resolution. Immunosuppressive agents have been used, but experience is limited.

157 An HIV-positive African patient has a CD4 count of 0.25×10^9/l and auramine-positive organisms in the bronchoscopic lavage fluid.

i. What does the chest radiograph (157) show and what is the likely diagnosis?

ii. How well does this condition respond to therapy?

iii. Can this disease be prevented?

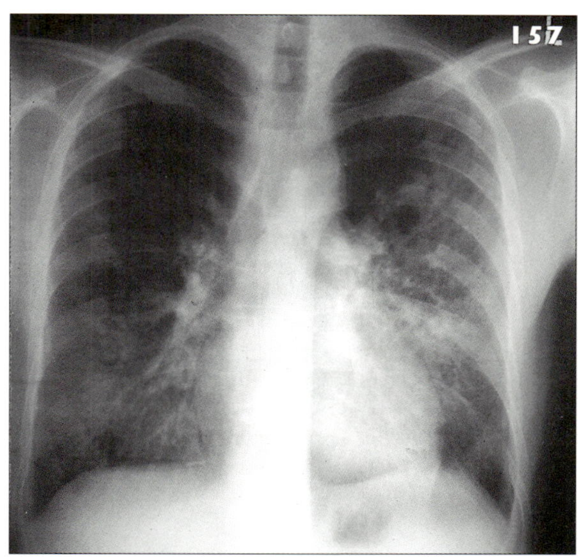

158 This optic fundus (158) of a 40-year-old woman who presented with bilateral facial palsy of sudden onset and also complained of headache and sore eyes.

i. Which multisystem disorder is the likely diagnosis?

ii. What other neurological manifestations occur in this disease?

iii. Comment on the sore eyes.

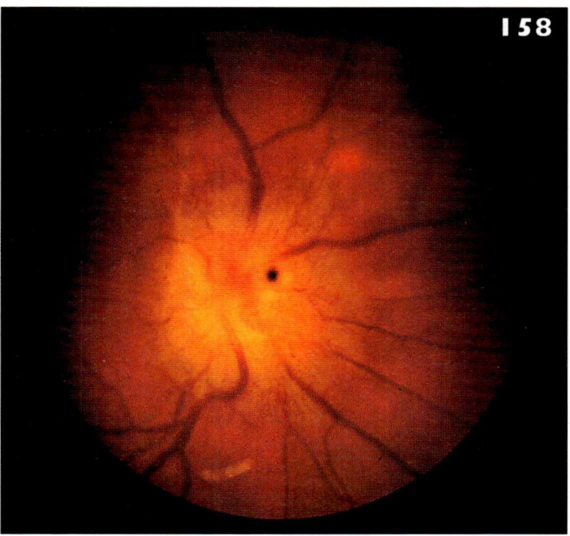

157 i. Patchy shadowing of the right lower zone and the left mid- and upper zones with large nodules on the left. Tuberculosis is the most likely cause given the patient's ethnic origin and the relatively high CD4 lymphocyte count.

ii. Treatment with standard triple or quadruple anti-tuberculous drug regimens (see below) bring about radiographic and microbiological improvement at the same rate as in HIV-negative patients, providing the organism is sensitive to the antibiotics. There is a high mortality rate, both during and soon after therapy, from other HIV-related causes. Drug-resistant strains of *M. tuberculosis* are present in developing countries and in developed countries such as New York and Miami in the USA. Patients from areas where drug resistance is common should commence therapy with four drugs (usually rifampicin, isoniazid, pyrazinamide and ethambutol). Patients with fully sensitive organisms need be treated for 6 months only, whereas with resistance therapy with second-line drugs should be given for 9–12 months.

iii. Primary chemoprophylaxis with isoniazid given for 12 months will benefit certain HIV-positive patients namely: tuberculin-positive (>4 mm Mantoux reaction) individuals from countries or groups (e.g. intravenous drug users) with a prevalence of tuberculosis greater than 10%. Tuberculin-negative patients from these areas who show anergy on skin testing with other antigens will also benefit from primary isoniazid prophylaxis. Secondary prophylaxis (long-term therapy with isoniazid following successful treatment of tuberculosis) is recommended by the British and American Thoracic Societies.

158 i. This woman has raised intracranial pressure with papilloedema from neurosarcoidosis which has caused her facial palsies. She has meningeal involvement with increased CSF pressure, a mild lymphocytic pleocytosis and increased protein but without meningeal symptoms. Papilloedema can also be caused by direct involvement of the optic nerve as well as by space-occupying masses of sarcoid tissue. Facial paresis, either unilateral or bilateral is the most common CNS manifestation.

ii. Involvement of the occulomotor, trochlear and abducens nerves are rare. Trigeminal sensory loss, sensorineural hearing loss and vertigo are fairly common. The most common abnormality of the peripheral nerves is a symmetrical peripheral neuropathy, although scattered patchy sensory neuropathies are also common. Motor involvement is less common and should not be confused with chronic sarcoid myopathy.

iii. About 25% of patients have some form of eye involvement. Sarcoid involvement of the lacrimal and salivary glands is very common and causes a sicca syndrome with dry mouth and sore, gritty eyes which may mimic Sjögren's syndrome. Artificial tears and saliva are useful. Anterior uveitis is the most frequent ocular finding which occurs more in commonly in blacks, the acute form (iridocyclitis) causing a painful, red eye with photophobia and blurred vision. Posterior uveitis occurs more commonly in whites and can cause visual loss from neovascularization. Fluorescein angiography is useful for demonstrating sarcoid retinitis. A slit lamp examination should be done in all patients with sarcoidosis and a Schirmer's test to assess lacrimation.

159 i. Name the systemic disease that most likely accounts for the findings seen in **159a** and **159b**.
ii. Name six pleuropulmonary manifestations of this disease.
iii. Characterize the expecting findings from a thoracentesis of a pleural effusion that has occurred as a result of this disease.

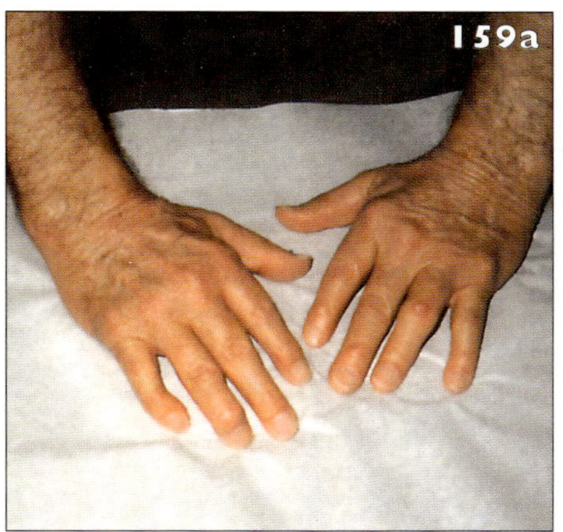

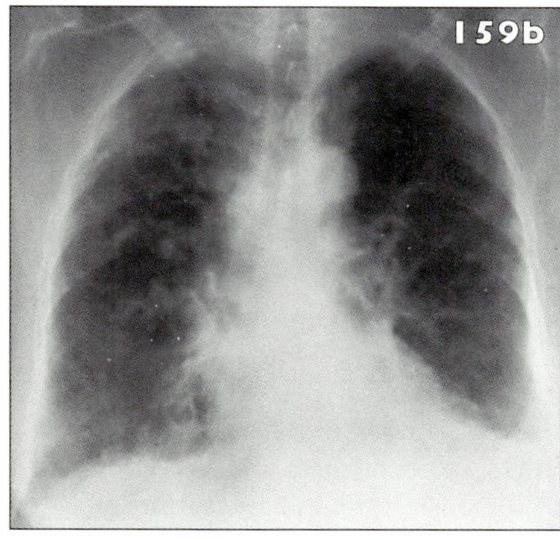

160 i. What is the differential diagnosis of daytime hypersomnolence?
ii. How would the history help in differentiating these diagnoses?

161 When this patient (**161**), who has a CD4 lymphocyte count of 0.15×10^9/l, became ill several weeks previously with malaise and subcutaneous swellings, lymphadenopathy was the primary finding. Investigations for mycobacteria were negative. He now complains of dyspnoea of 2 days' duration and is hypoxic at rest.
i. What is the probable cause of his respiratory symptoms?
ii. List the possible causes of the mediastinal widening. How may the cause be confirmed?

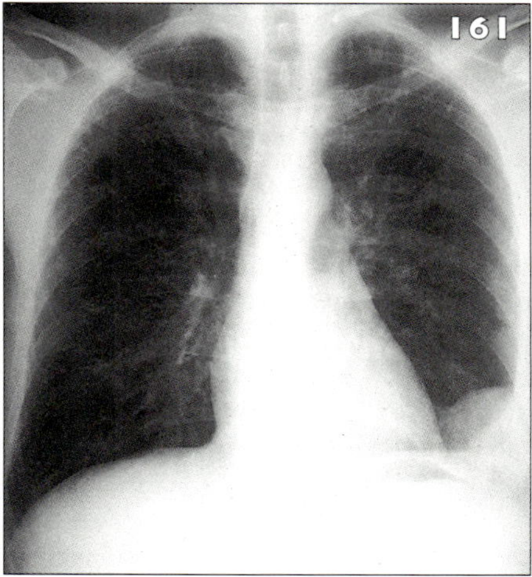

159 i. Rheumatoid arthritis is the most likely diagnosis. The hands (**159a**) depict ulnar deviation, characteristic in this disorder. The chest radiograph (**159b**) findings include the presence of pleural effusions and interstitial fibrosis. The basal and peripheral distribution of the shadowing is characteristic of fibrosing alveolitis; and the lung parenchymal pathology and management is identical to that for cryptogenic fibrosing alveolitis (CFA).

ii. The pleuropulmonary manifestations of rheumatoid arthritis include pleural effusions, diffuse interstitial pneumonitis and fibrosis, necrobiotic rheumatoid nodules, Caplan's syndrome (rheumatoid pneumoconiosis), obliterative bronchiolitis and pulmonary vasculitis. Pleural disease is the most common intrathoracic manifestation – vasculitis affecting the pulmonary vasculature is exceptionally rare.

iii. Pleural fluid of patients with rheumatoid arthritis is characteristically exudative (protein >30 g/l), and the cellular component is predominantly lymphocytic. The glucose content may be exceedingly low (e.g. <30 mg/dl) even in the absence of infection. Rheumatoid factor titres can be very high.

160 i. The differential diagnosis includes: intrinsic causes such as obstructive sleep apnoea, narcolepsy, idiopathic hypersomnia, post-traumatic hypersomnia, periodic movements of the legs/restless sleep and extrinsic causes such as poor 'sleep hygiene', insufficient sleep, hypnotic/sedative abuse and alcohol abuse.

ii. In obstructive sleep apnoea, there is a history of steady progression of symptoms, often over many years. Initially there is snoring which becomes more pronounced, turning into periods of apnoea and restlessness which becomes more numerous and prolonged. This is noted by the partner rather than the patient. It develops fully by middle age, is more common in men and is associated with weight gain, increased alcohol intake and night sedation. In classical narcolepsy there is a history of cataplexy and at least one of the other three symptoms: sleepiness, sleep paralysis and hypnagogic hallucinations. In periodic leg movement there is an irresistible urge to move the legs, causing insomnia and sleep disruption. In post-traumatic hypersomnia, there is a history of preceding head injury, stroke or brain surgery .

161 i. Any acute respiratory illness such as this should be considered to be PCP until proven otherwise. The differential diagnosis is bacterial pneumonia, tuberculosis, histoplasmosis (in endemic areas) and pulmonary oedema due to left ventricular failure. Infections with atypical mycobacteria, *C. neoformans* and cytomegalovirus are less likely given that the CD4 count is above 0.1×10^9/l. PCP does not explain the pleural shadow.

ii. Given his history of recent onset generalized lymphadenopathy, the pleural pathology is likely to be caused by the same pathology, and include mycobacterial infection, lymphoma, Kaposi's sarcoma and cryptococcal infection. The diagnosis in this patient (lymphoma) would be confirmed by lymph-node biopsy from one of the subcutaneous lesions. If there are no suitable subcutaneous nodes, the cause in this case may be found by biopsying the pleural mass. Lymphoma might also be found on bone marrow biopsy although the diagnostic yield of this procedure is low.

162 Shown in **162a** is the radiograph of a previously fit 42-year-old woman who was seen in the emergency department with a 36-hour history of a flu-like illness and increasing respiratory compromise. Her fingers and nailbeds shortly after admission to intensive care are shown in **162b**.
i. What would be the factors that you would take into consideration when deciding whether to admit this patient with pneumonia to the intensive therapy unit?
ii. Which complications are suggested by **162b**?

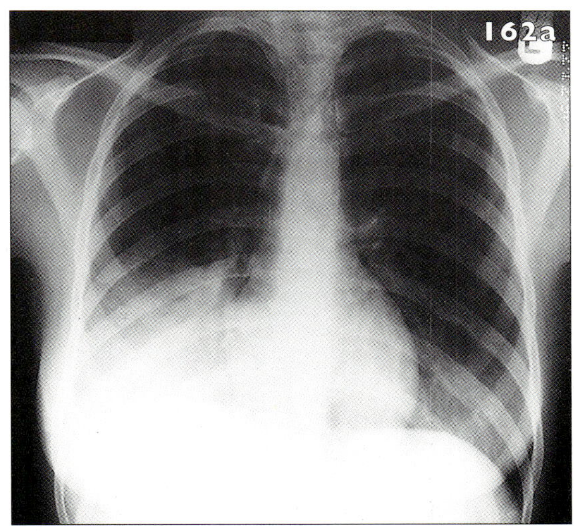

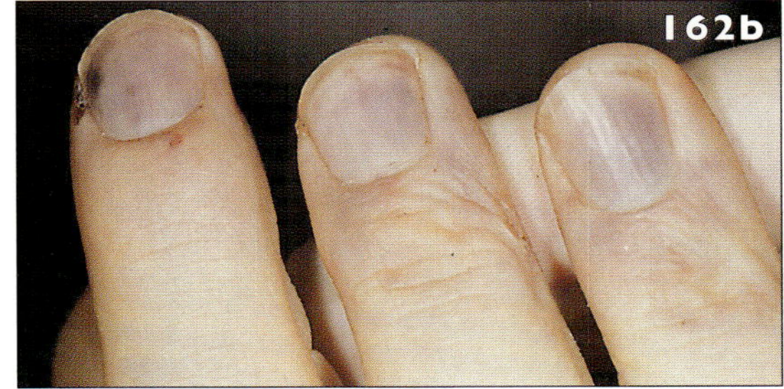

163 A previously healthy athletic 32-year-old male has worked in this environment (**163**) for 3 years. Over the past several months he has experienced worsening nocturnal chest tightness and wheezing.
i. What is the differential diagnosis?
ii. What are risk factors for occupational asthma?
iii. What is the likely antigen in this case?
iv. Should the patient be advised to seek other work? Why?

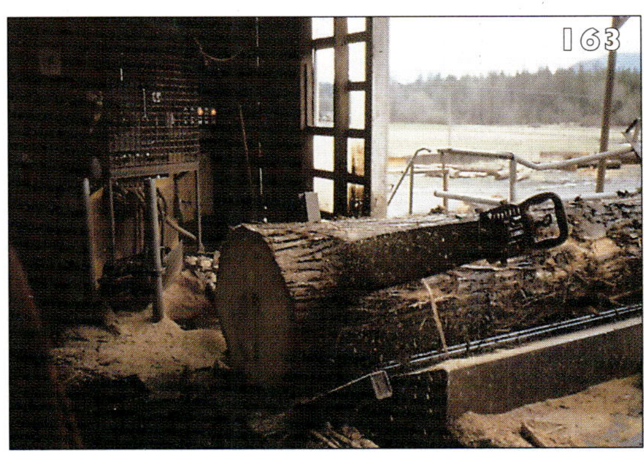

162 i. The chest radiograph (**162a**) shows right lower lobe consolidation and, in a previously fit 42-year-old woman, the most likely causative organism is the pneumococcus. From the British Thoracic Society Guidelines on community-acquired pneumonia, the features associated with an increased risk of death are (** indicates strongest association):

- **Clinical:** (a) respiratory rate >30/minute**; (b) diastolic BP <60 mmHg**; (c) age >60 years; (d) confusion; (e) atrial fibrillation; (f) multi-lobar involvement; (g) underlying disease.
- **Laboratory:** (a) serum urea >7 mmol/l**; (b) serum albumin <35 g/l; (c) PaO_2 <8 kPa (60 mmHg); (d) WBC<4000 or >20 000 $x10^9/l$.

ii. The photograph of the fingers/nailbeds shows peripheral cyanosis and a distal vascular infarct. Although the limb peripheries may be cold and poorly perfused the global systemic vascular resistance is frequently low, emphasizing the marked variation in regional vascular tone that typifies sepsis. While it is important to ensure that the intravascular volume is adequate and some colloid infusion may be necessary, this should neither be excessive nor administered too rapidly if deterioration in pulmonary gas exchange and marked tissue oedema are to be avoided. The infarct may be a thrombotic manifestation of disseminated intravascular coagulation (DIC) a frequent complication of severe pneumococcal pneumonia

163 i. Bronchial hyperreactivity and airflow limitation associated with occupational asthma, non-occupational asthma, gastro-oesophageal reflux, and posterior nasal drip may present with nocturnal chest tightness and wheezing. Acute extrinsic allergic alveolitis (or hypersensitivity pneumonitis) should be considered but usually presents with prominent constitutional symptoms of fever, chills and myalgias in addition to cough, dyspnoea and chest tightness.

ii. More than 200 agents have been implicated in occupational asthma. High-molecular weight sensitizers (i.e. >1000 kDa) such as proteins and polysaccharides typically produce an immediate asthmatic reaction through IgE-mediated mechanisms. Atopy and smoking are risk factors. Low-molecular weight compounds (<1000 kDa) are associated with an isolated late asthmatic response occurring 4 to 12 h after exposure. A biphasic response with early and late reductions in expiratory flow with intervening recovery or a prolonged early response may also occur. Non-atopic individuals are affected more commonly.

iii. Western red cedar (*Thuja plicata*) is widely used for shakes, shingles and lumber in North America. Plicatic acid (440 kDa) is the primary sensitizer in red cedar asthma. Nocturnal cough, wheeze and chest tightness are characteristic presenting features.

iv. Eliminating exposure to the antigen is the primary therapy for occupational asthma. Asthma persists in 60% of affected workers, even after leaving the industry.

164 i. What medications can be used to treat OSA?
ii. Patients with OSA should have what additional abnormality before being considered candidates for progestational agents?

165 This high-resolution CT scan (**165**) of a 30-year-old man with sarcoidosis showing a reticulonodular pattern.
i. What is the advantage of HRCT over conventional CT?
ii. Describe the HRCT findings in sarcoidosis.
iii. When would you do a HRCT?

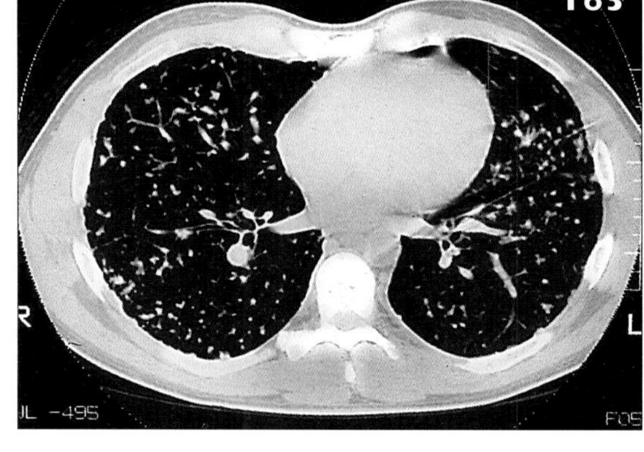

166 A 25-year-old Asian Indian man presents with fevers, cough and weight loss over 3 months; **166b** was taken four months after **166a**.
i. What is the likely diagnosis?
ii. Enumerate the abnormalities on the chest radiographs.
iii. How quickly and to what extent will these changes improve with treatment?

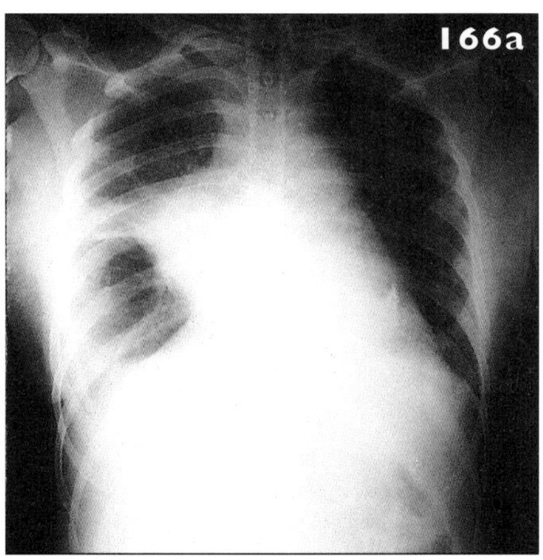
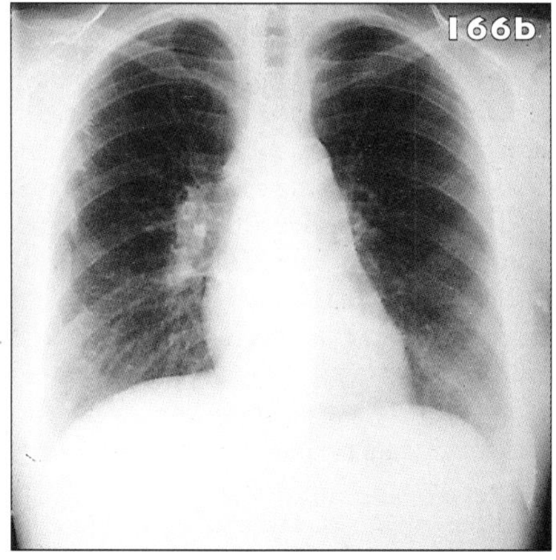

164 i. The role of drugs in the management of OSA is limited. Protriptyline, a tricyclic antidepressant, has been shown to reduce sleepiness, improve nocturnal oxygenation and decrease apnoea frequency in patients with OSA by reducing the proportion of total sleep time spent in REM. Since apnoeas tend to be more frequent and severe during REM sleep, this tends to improve oxygenation and the frequency of sleep-disordered breathing. It has also been proposed that protriptyline augments the activity of upper airway dilator muscles. The clinical utility of protriptyline remains small.

ii. Progestational agents have no role in the treatment of eucapnic patients with OSA. They may have a role in treating hypercapnic patients with sleep-disordered breathing, in particular those with obesity hypoventilation syndrome, though this may be due to its effects on alveolar hypoventilation rather than sleep-disordered breathing. A beneficial effect in reducing sleep-disordered breathing (either central or obstructive) in hypercapnic individuals has not been demonstrated specifically.

165 i. HRCT gives outstanding definition of the lung parenchyma by taking rapid thin slices (1–2 mm). Conventional CT takes 8–10-mm slices and is therefore less useful for small nodules and more subtle abnormalities.

ii. The characteristic parenchymal abnormalities of sarcoidosis are small nodular densities along the lymphatics, particularly the bronchovascular bundles and interlobular septae. Subpleural nodules are also very common. A hazy ground-glass appearance (alveolar filling), although uncommon, is usually associated with severe dyspnoea and hypoxia. Other features seen include linear opacities, end-stage fibrosis and cysts, traction bronchiectasis and honey-comb lung.

iii. Sometimes with more patchy and focal sarcoidosis HRCT can be useful to guide the bronchoscopist performing transbronchial biopsies. HRCT may show severe diffuse alveolar disease not obvious on chest radiography, but it has a limited role. It cannot be recommended as a routine screening tool or to assess response to treatment.

166 i. Tuberculosis is the likely diagnosis.

ii. The abnormalities include a large right hilar mass. There is opacification of the right upper lobe probably due to bronchial narrowing by the hilar nodal mass. There is also cardiomegaly, possibly due to pericardial effusion.

iii. The second radiograph (**166b**) was taken 2 months after starting standard four-drug anti-tuberculous chemotherapy and shows significant resolution with only residual right hilar shadowing. Improvement had started after 1 month. In monitoring for the effects of TB treatment lack of radiographic improvement by 2 months may mean either the changes are chronic or there is a problem with therapy, usually due to non-compliance. However, the changes seen on the chest radiograph are not a good predictor of response to treatment. Radiographic improvement is usually complete by 6 months, although some patients continue to improve for 12 months. However, the most important sign of improvement is sputum smears and culture becoming negative; failure here means the disease has not been eradicated.

167 An elderly woman complained of shortness of breath on exertion but was otherwise in good health.
i. What abnormalities are evident on the chest radiograph (**167a**) and CT film (**167b**) and what is the likely diagnosis?
ii. What further diagnostic tests are likely to be of value?
iii. What risks are associated with this condition?
iv. What management is advisable and what specific risks should be mentioned to the patient?

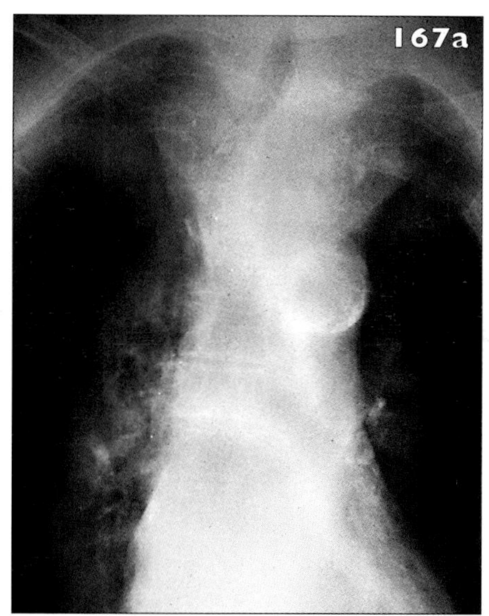

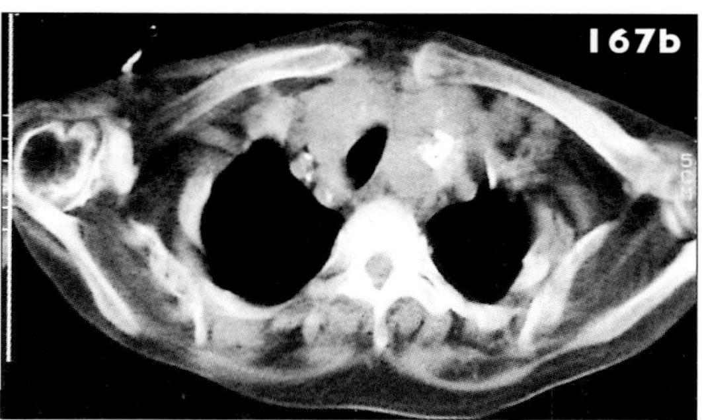

168 Describe the important aspects of good sleep hygiene.

169 A 60-year-old man complained of increasing back and left-sided chest pain for approximately 6 months. What does the scan (**169**) show and how would you confirm the diagnosis?

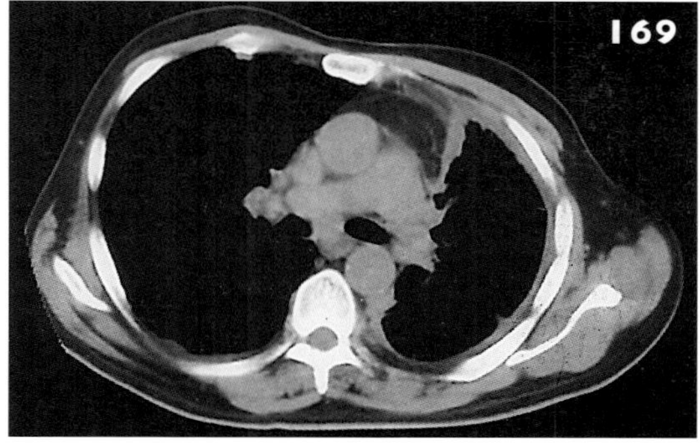

167 i. There is an upper mediastinal mass which exhibits areas of calcification (poorly seen on radiograph). The trachea is markedly deviated. The features are those of a retrosternal thyroid goitre.
ii. None. Radio-iodine scanning is frequently performed but is almost never of value as the goitre will not take up the iodine. Bronchoscopy is non-contributory. Needle biopsy might reveal a thyroid carcinoma but this would be unlikely to exhibit calcification and a negative core would not exclude this diagnosis.
iii. Any airway obstruction can worsen with deteriorating exercise tolerance. Haemorrhage can occur into the gland causing acute enlargement and an airway emergency. Malignant degeneration has been reported very rarely.
iv. Subtotal thyroidectomy is indicated to relieve airway compression. This is usually possible through a collar incision. The chief hazards are damage to the recurrent laryngeal nerves and transient postoperative hypocalcaemia from parathyroid injury. Very occasionally, tracheomalacia may exist which results in instability of the tracheal wall postoperatively and difficulty with respiration.

168 Diagnosing and treating sleep problems requires knowledge of good sleep hygiene. Recommendations can be divided into broad categories:
- Encouraging normal homeostatic and circadian rhythms. The patient should maintain regular bedtime and arising times. Naps should generally be avoided but if necessary be limited to 20 minutes . Daily exercise in the morning or afternoon is helpful. A warm bath 20–30 minutes before retiring can promote sleep.
- Maintaining a conducive sleep setting. The bedroom should be dark, quiet, well-ventilated and at a comfortable temperature. The mattress and pillows should be comfortable. The bedroom should be only used for sleep and sex, not for other activities which require prolonged arousal. Avoid heavy snacking or drinking just before bedtime.
- Avoiding drugs that interfere with sleep. Tobacco, caffeine, and alcohol should be avoided within several hours of sleep.

169 Malignant pleural mesothelioma without effusion. The scan (**169**) shows gross irregular pleural thickening, with characteristic constriction of that hemithorax. Approximately 30% of malignant pleural mesotheliomas present as either diffuse pleural thickening or as a localized pleural mass without significant effusion. Thoracoscopy is impossible in these cases as the pleural cavity is often obliterated. The diagnosis can usually be confirmed by CT-guided needle biopsy. Thoracotomy should be avoided. Pain is often severe and intractable and neurolytic procedures, such as cervical cordotomy, may be necessary for its control.

Most patients with mesothelioma recall significant exposure to asbestos. The greater the exposure the higher the chance of developing this complication. About 30% of cases have no history of any contact with asbestos, confirming that this tumour has other causes – as yet not known. Other inorganic fibres such as tremolite, which occurs naturally in the soil in some countries (for example Cyprus), can also cause mesothelioma.

170 Shown is a high-power photomicrograph (**170**) of the Gram stain of sputum expectorated by a 19-year-old man with symptoms of fever, rigors and a productive cough of 2 days' duration. He has experienced four episodes of radiographically documented pneumonia and numerous episodes of acute otitis media and sinusitis in the past.

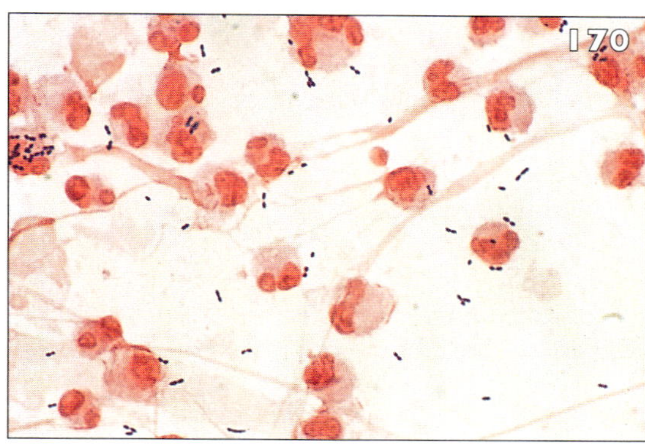

i. What does the Gram stain show?
ii. What is the most likely diagnosis?
iii. What additional the diagnostic considerations are raised by this clinical presentation?

171 A patient presents with a 2-week history of progressive weakness of the arms and shoulders, difficulty in swallowing and a dry mouth. The chest radiograph (**171**) shows a mass in the right paratracheal region.
i. What is the likely diagnosis of this presentation?
ii. How would you make the diagnosis?
iii. How would you treat the patient?

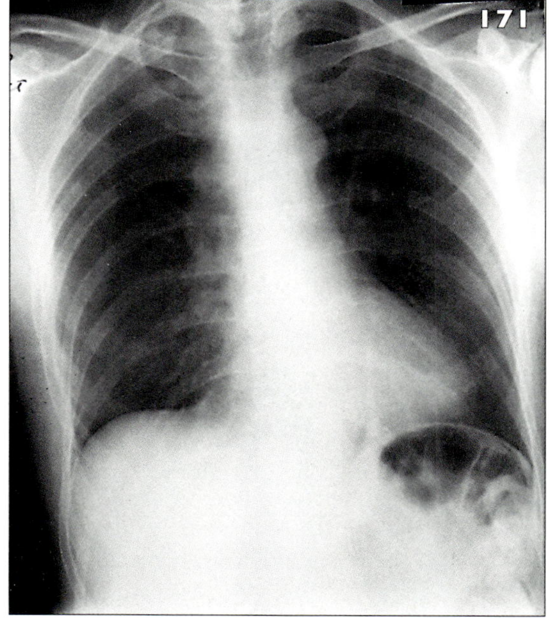

170 i. The sputum Gram stain (170) shows numerous polymorphonuclear leukocytes, strands of mucus, and many Gram-positive, lancet-shaped diplococci. Refractile capsules are evident on many of the bacteria.
ii. This young patient has an acute pneumococcal pneumonia and has suffered numerous recurrent respiratory infections.
iii. Most patients with recurrent respiratory infections have no identifiable host defect. However, recurrent pneumonias in the same lobe or segment should suggest an anatomical abnormality. When multiple sites have been involved, disorders of mucociliary clearance such as cystic fibrosis or the ciliary dyskinesia syndrome (Kartagener's syndrome) are important considerations. Recurrent infections with encapsulated organisms such as the pneumococcus are consistent with a defect in opsonization (e.g. complement, IgG or IgG subtype deficiencies). Deficiencies of complement components are rare and are best managed by immunization and by early treatment of infectious complications. Immunoglobulin deficiencies also can be primary (inherited), or acquired due to acquired B-cell disorders, medications or intercurrent illnesses. IgA is heavily concentrated in mucosal secretions where it inhibits bacterial adherence. Although selective IgA deficiency is common, it rarely results in serious respiratory infection unless other deficiencies coexist. IgG deficiency (either generalized or restricted to subclasses IgG1 and IgG3) predisposes to more frequent and to more severe respiratory infections. Intravenous immunoglobulin replacement may be helpful.

171 i. The chest radiograph (171) shows paratracheal lymphadenopathy likely due to a malignant tumour. The patient has a myopathy and the difficulty in swallowing and dry mouth is suggestive of the Lambert–Eaton syndrome (LEMS). The tendon reflexes will be absent, but will become present after repetitive forced contraction of the relevant muscle group. Repeated short-term use of muscle groups will also increase their strength temporarily. An EMG will show post-tetanic potentiation.
ii. LEMS is a para-malignant syndrome strongly associated with small-cell lung cancer. It may precede the clinical appearance of a tumour by many months. The diagnosis is made by the diagnosis of SCLC, the neurological physical signs and the response of the tendon jerks to muscle activity and the characteristic findings on EMG.
iii. Treatment is both specifically aimed at the LEMS and also, more generally, at the primary tumour.

Specific treatment for LEMS is high dose corticosteroids, e.g. prednisolone 60 mg daily, and 3–4 mg/day aminopyridine, which is an anti-cholinergic antagonist. Resolution of the tumour will provide the greatest symptomatic benefit and the best chance of remission. The syndrome can show considerable improvement with resolution of the primary tumour, but recurrence of the syndrome usually heralds relapse.

172 A patient presents with bilateral hilar lymphadenopathy and parenchymal infiltrates. A diagnosis of sarcoidosis is made. There is no other active organ involvement. What is the role if any of oral corticosteroids (OCS) in this case?

173 Fever, cough and dyspnoea were the presenting features of this man's illness (**173a**). His CD4+ lymphocyte count is 0.08×10^9/l.
i. Describe the cytological finding in the bronchoalveolar lavage (BAL) specimen (**173b**) and give the diagnosis of his condition.
ii. What is a more common presentation of disease caused by this agent?
iii. Discuss the management of this condition and any potential complications.

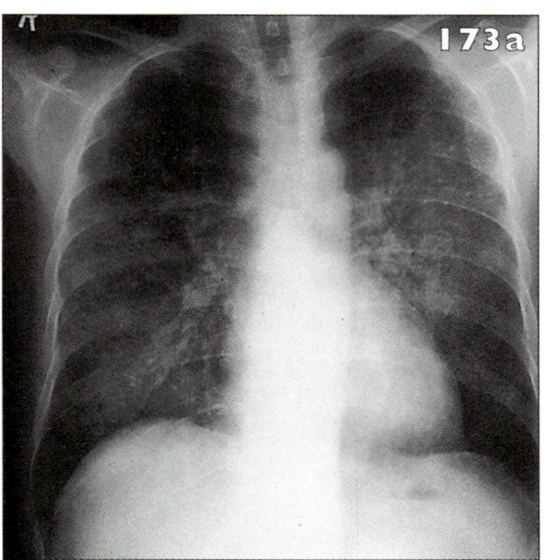

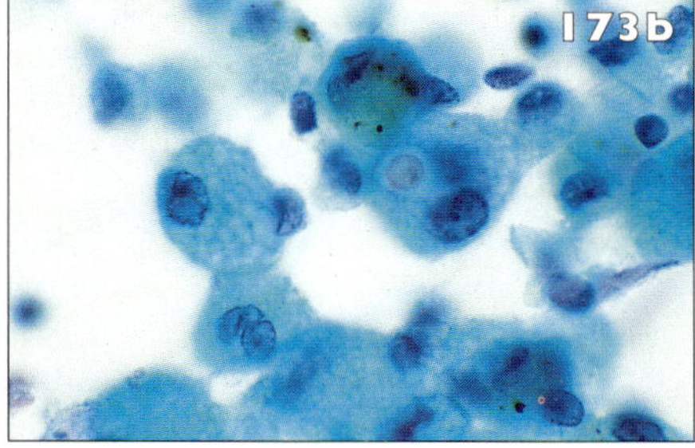

174 This patient whose upper trachea is shown (**174**) underwent tracheostomy for prolonged mechanical ventilation 6 months previously. Breathlessness is now occurring.
i. What has occurred?
ii. How is this managed?

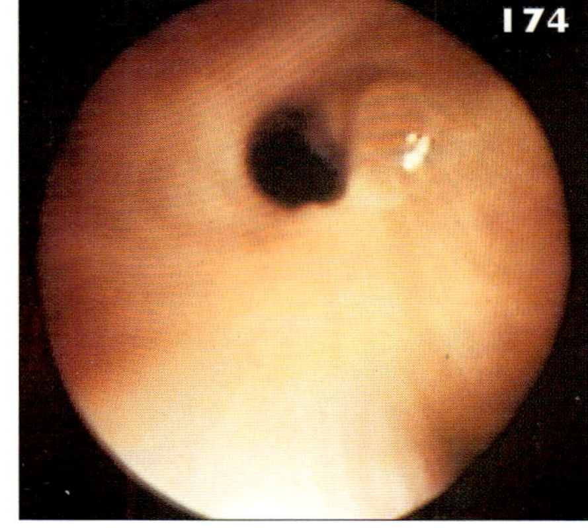

172 i. A recent study by the British Thoracic Society has helped to clarify the role of OCS in pulmonary involvement by sarcoidosis. If the symptoms and functional measurements are deteriorating, then OCS should be commenced at a dose of 40 mg per day for 1 month, then slowly reduced. The majority of such patients will improve on therapy, although relapse is common on reducing or stopping the steroids. If the condition remains stable when untreated, the addition of OCS for at least 18 months will produce small improvements in the radiographic and functional measurements compared with no treatment, but the advantage of treating stable disease is small and will inevitably be associated with some steroid-related side effects. It is still not clear whether OCS affect the long-term outcome in sarcoidosis but it seems reasonable to treat patients whose condition is deteriorating during the first 6 months of the clinical course.

173 i. This encapsulated intracellular yeast is typical of *Cryptococcus neoformans*. This can be confirmed by antigen testing of the blood and culture of blood and BAL fluid. Other yeasts that cause lung disease include *Candida* sp. and *Histoplasma capsulatum*, but these can be distinguished on morphology and culture.
ii. A sub-acute meningitis would be the most common presentation of illness caused by this organism in AIDS.
iii. Cryptococcal infection is treated with intravenous amphotericin B, sometimes with the addition of flucytosine, in more severe cases. Alternatively, fluconazole (orally or intravenously) is used for less severe cases. High-dose treatment is given for 4–6 weeks, followed by long-term secondary prophylaxis – usually with oral fluconazole. Treatment response is usually monitored by clinical parameters and falling cryptococcal antigen titres. Respiratory disease may lead to respiratory failure and meningitis can progress to widespread involvement of the brain (cryptococcomas) and hydrocephalus.

174 i. A post-tracheostomy tracheal stricture.
ii. Definitive management in symptomatic patients is surgical resection of the involved tracheal segment. The maximum length of trachea that can be resected is 50%, i.e. about 5–6 cm. In cases where there is acute breathlessness, temporizing measures include YAG laser resection to widen the orifice. Laser treatment may be particularly useful in preventing surgery if the patient is still recovering from their initial illness. Best results are obtained when the stricture is primarily mucosal and does not have extensive fibrosis of the tracheal wall. In the unusual case of a long segment of stenosis, tracheal stenting may be used. Non-metal stents are deployed so that they may be removed at a later date. Prolonged stenting occasionally causes a stricture usually more than a year after placement. With the increasing use of percutaneous tracheostomy performed in intensive care units this complication of tracheostomy may decline.

175 Pleural biopsies from two patients with large pleural effusions are shown in **175a** and **175b**. The reported differential diagnosis for both was adenocarcinoma and mesothelioma.
i. How can the two be differentiated?
ii. Why is it important to make this distinction?
iii. Should primary sites be looked for in cases of metastatic pleural adenocarcinoma?

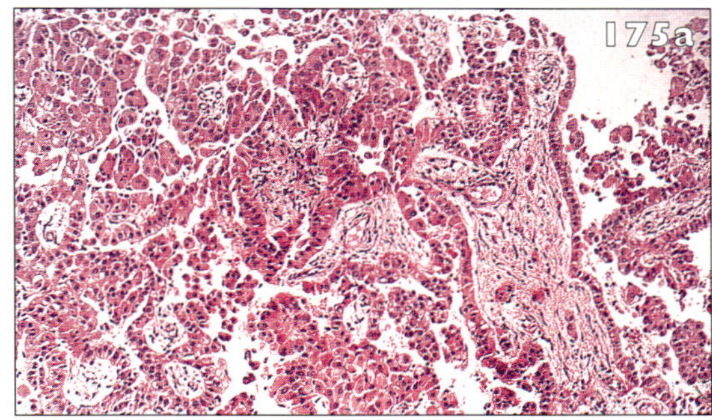

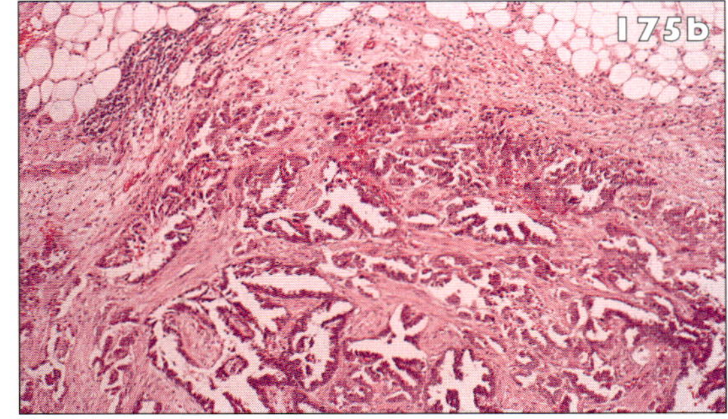

176 This is the chest radiograph (**176a**) of a 65-year-old man, a 40 pack year smoker.
i. What is the likely diagnosis?
ii. What investigations are necessary to stage the patient?
iii. What is the treatment of choice?

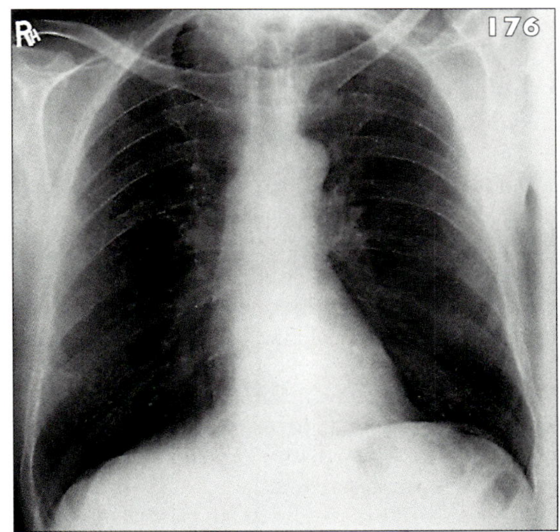

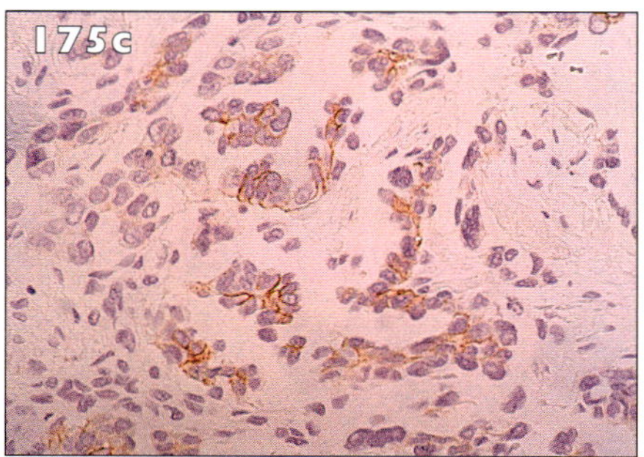

175 i. 175b shows papillary and glandular structures and 175a also shows glandular structures, making distinction between the two difficult. 175b was also stained for AUA 1 (175c) and was positive, which is specific for adenocarcinoma. Staining of the other biopsy (175a) was negative suggesting mesothelioma. Positive confirmation of mesothelioma is more difficult and requires the use of electron microscopy.

ii. Confirmation of a diagnosis of mesothelioma is very important for patients with documented asbestos exposure who wish to pursue compensation claims.

iii. No survival advantage has been shown in pursuing the primary site of adenocarcinomas in these patients. The most common site is the lung itself, followed by breast and gastrointestinal tumours.

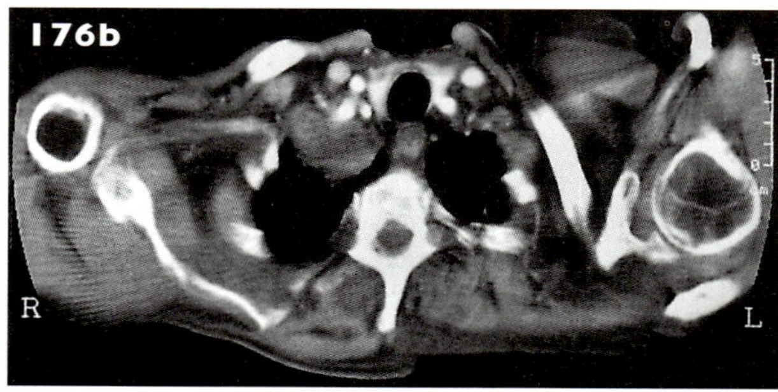

176 i. The lesion in the right apex has a 95% chance of being a primary carcinoma of the bronchus in a man of this age and smoking history. The irregular margins seen first on CT (176b) make a malignant lesion probable. Benign lesions would be smoother as would a solitary metastasis.

ii. The lesion ideally should be removed. A fine-needle aspiration is not useful as it will either confirm what one suspects, and is unlikely to be diagnostic if the lesion is benign. A pneumothorax following a needle biopsy may 'soil' the pleura and increase the risk of postoperative infection. A CT scan of the thorax and upper abdomen is the investigation of choice. Nodal enlargement in the mediastinum needs to be excluded. If present, mediastinoscopy should be performed to confirm or exclude metastatic nodal spread. The CT will also confirm whether the lesion is solitary. There is no benefit in performing a fibre-optic bronchoscopy as it is unlikely to yield a diagnosis or any new information.

iii. The treatment of choice is a thoracotomy. A frozen section of the lesion is mandatory as benign disease requires no more than enucleation or a segmental resection. A primary tumour should be removed by lobectomy. If lung function is poor, then segmentectomy can be performed, but the 5-year survival is not as good as for lobectomy, which is in the region of 50–70% for a stage I lesion, i.e. solitary with no hilar or mediastinal nodal involvement.

177 A 34-year-old woman in otherwise excellent health presented with a non-specific cough. Chest film (**177a**) and CT scan (**177b**) demonstrated a cystic lesion in the mediastinum.
i. What is your differential diagnosis?
ii. What treatment is indicated and why?
iii. What specific difficulties may surgery present?

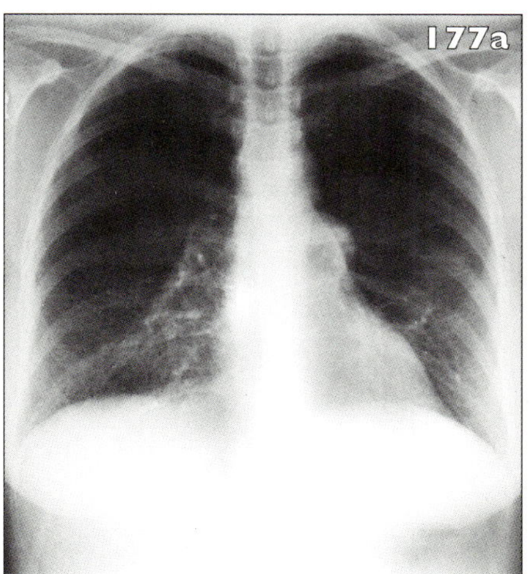
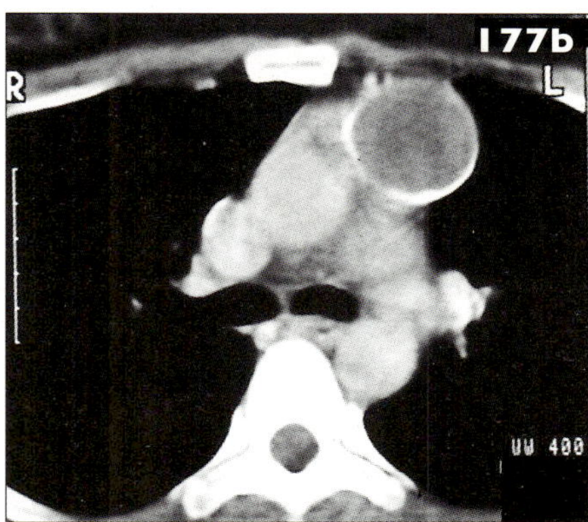

178 i. How does the small hole in the nebulizer base allow jet nebulizing to occur (**178a, 178b**)?
ii. What parameters of flow rate and nebulizer volume are most effective?
iii. What percentage of nebulized solution will be deposited in the lungs?

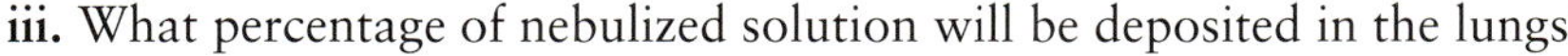
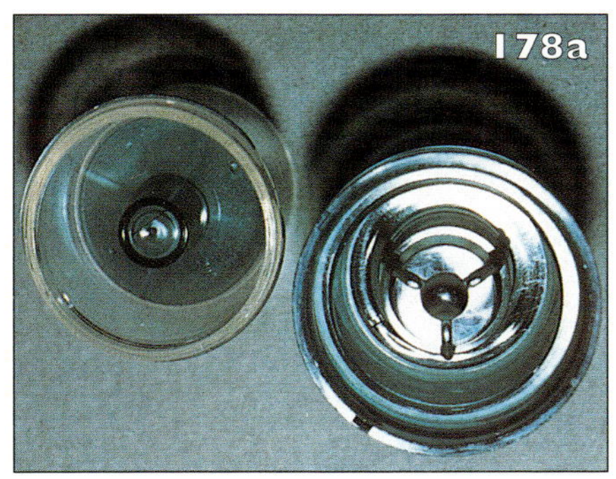
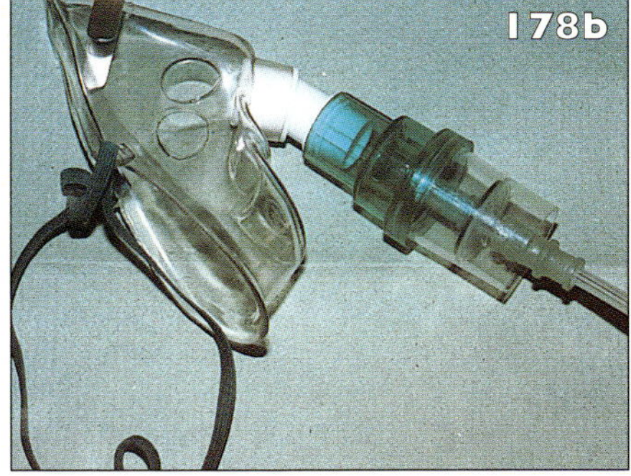

177 i. This lesion is located in the anterior compartment. It is fluid-filled and has a thick, calcified wall suggesting a benign origin. The most likely possibility is, therefore, a dermoid cyst. A thymic cyst would usually have a much thinner wall. In the relevant countries, echinococcus would have to be considered. Pleuropericardial cysts arise posterior to the anterior edge of the pericardium.

ii. The likely benign nature would suggest that a policy of observation would be satisfactory in the elderly or infirm. There exists, however, the concern that the true diagnosis is uncertain unless the lesion is excised. There are also reports of these medastinal cysts eroding into a great vessel or becoming infected and rupturing into the pericardium. In most cases it is usual to advise excision of the lesion.

Note : In this case the lesion is cystic and a benign germ cell cyst is suspected. Had the lesion been solid, a malignant germ cell lesion would have to be considered, particularly in young males. Alpha-fetoprotein and beta-HCG should be measured. Elevated levels are encountered in all non-seminomatous-type tumours and in about 10% of mediastinal seminomas. Excision or biopsy is undertaken in this situation depending upon resectability. Chemotherapy should be given and radiotherapy to the mediastinum is also indicated for seminomas.

iii. Adhesions can be dense around dermoid cysts and in extreme cases it may be necessary to excise a portion of the cyst and 'deroof' it rather than excise the whole lesion.

178 i. As the driving gas (either oxygen or compressed air) enters the hole a jet is created. Liquid contained in the base of the nebulizer is drawn upward in a funnel towards the jet and drawn into it by the Bernoulli effect. As the jet hits the baffles above it (**178b**), larger particles are removed, their size depending on the characteristics of the baffles. Deposition of particles >10 μm may occur in the oropharynx, those of 5–10 μm in the tracheobronchial tree, and those of 2–5 μm reach the alveoli. Factors other than particle size affect pattern of deposition, including the effect of airway humidity, evaporation, and particle agglomeration.

ii. Approximately 1 ml of solution is usually left on the baffles or in the well of the nebulizer at the end of a treatment. As solvent evaporates during nebulization there is a proportionately high amount of active drug in this residual fluid. Some 4 ml of solution is needed to counteract this problem, to allow the majority of the active drug to be nebulized. The recommended flow rate is 6–8 l/min, which allows high nebulizer output and generates suitably sized respirable particles.

iii. About 12% of the drug will reach the lung, making this mode of delivery no more efficient than metered dose-aerosols, spacers or powders.

179 A woman complained of mild back ache. Her radiographs (**179a, 179b**) and CT (**179c**) were as shown.
i. What abnormality is present and what is the differential diagnosis?
ii. What further investigation may be helpful?

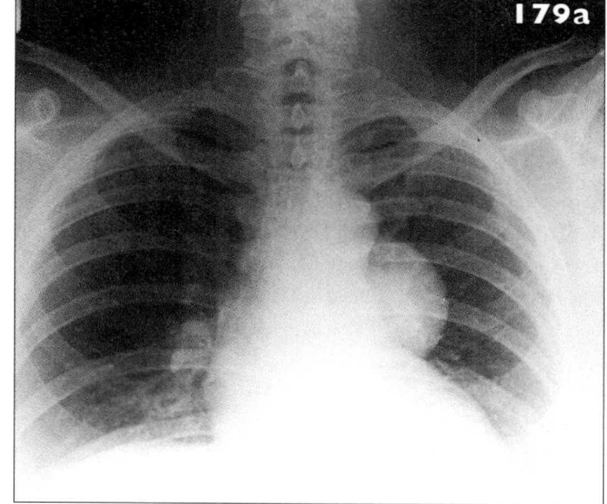

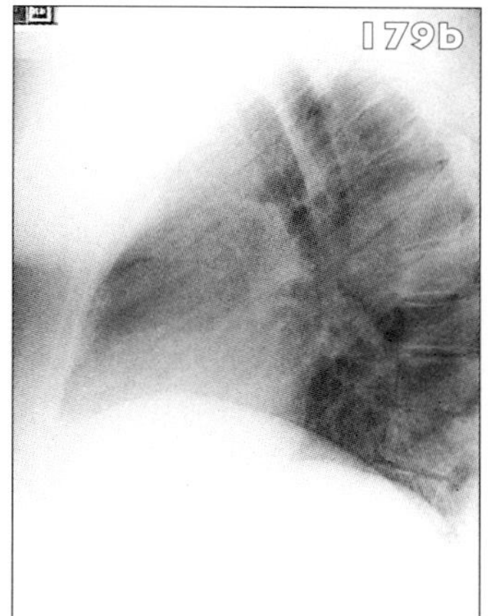

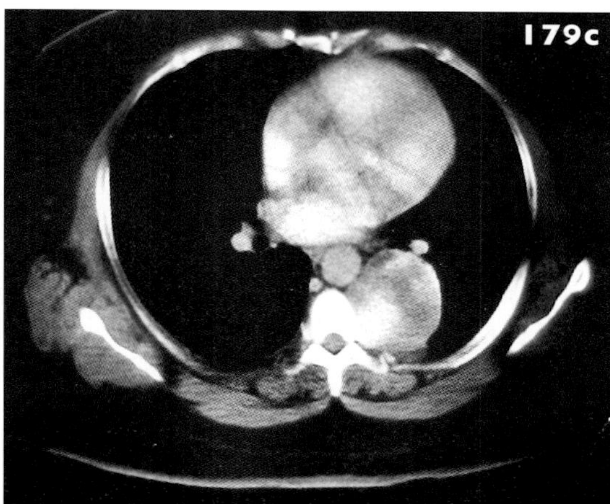

180 i. What are the presenting symptoms of narcolepsy?
ii. Which tests are useful in diagnosing narcolepsy?

179 i. A large mass is present in the left paravertebral sulcus adjacent to the vertebral column and rib heads. This position implies that the lesion is almost certainly a neurogenic tumour (**179a–c**). The differential most likely lies, therefore, between a neurilemmoma (schwannoma), neurofibroma or sarcoma (possibly in association with Von Recklinghausen's disease), ganglionoma and neuroblastoma. The simple neurilemmoma is much the most probable. Rarer possibilities in this site are: phaeochromocytoma, fibrosarcoma, lymphoma and mesenchymal tumours.
ii. It is important to establish whether a neural tumour extends into the vertebral canal and MRI may supplement CT scanning in determining this issue. An exterior mass can be excised at thoracotomy alone whereas a mass entering the vertebral foramen will require a combined approach with a neurosurgical team.

180 i. Unwanted episodes of sleep, daytime drowsiness, hypnagogic hallucinations, disturbed nocturnal sleep, cataplexy, and sleep paralysis are common symptoms of narcolepsy. Unwanted episodes of sleep can occur several times a day and in a variety of situations. Narcoleptics usually awaken refreshed from these episodes which can last from minutes to over one hour. Sleep onset can be accompanied by visual or auditory hypnagogic hallucinations. Cataplexy refers to an abrupt decrease in muscle tone which is often elicited by emotion. Cataplectic attacks can vary from a complete loss of muscle tone to a brief weakness of a particular muscle group. Sleep paralysis occurs at sleep onset or upon awakening. Patients find themselves unable to move, speak or open their eyes and often experience hallucinations. These episodes are usually less than 10 minutes in duration. Laser palatoplexy, which stiffens the uvula by inducing scar tissue, is probably as effective.
ii. HLA typing and Multiple Sleep Latency Testing (MSLT) are useful in the diagnosis of narcolepsy. An association between the major histocompatibility complex class II antigens DQw6 and Drw15 and narcolepsy has been established. DQw6 is the best current genetic marker and most, but not all, narcoleptics carry it. The MSLT consists of five or six scheduled naps during which the subject is monitored polygraphically in a dark, quiet bedroom. It is designed to measure physiological sleep tendencies in the absence of stimulating factors. Sleep latency and REM latency are measured. Mean sleep latencies less than 8 minutes are considered abnormal and consistent with excessive somnolence. REM sleep that occurs within 15 minutes of sleep onset is considered a sleep onset REM period. The presence of two or more sleep onset REM periods following a nocturnal polysomnogram which demonstrates normal sleep and the absence of other sleep disorders, supports the diagnosis of narcolepsy.

181 This chest radiograph (181) is from a 51-year-old man from south-east Asia with dyspnoea and leg swelling. He was jaundiced and had jugular venous distension and ascites on physical examination.
i. What are the radiographic findings?
ii. What infection could account for both the clinical and radiographic abnormalities?
iii. How can this diagnosis be established?
iv. How is it treated?

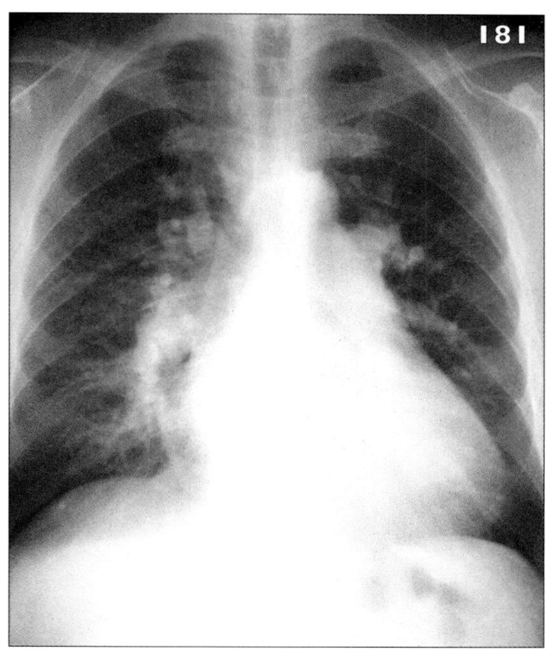

182 The chest radiograph (182) is from a 32-year-old female presenting with exertional dyspnoea.
i. What symptoms, physical findings and lung function abnormalities would you look for to confirm a diagnosis of idiopathic pulmonary fibrosis (IPF) associated with this disorder?
ii. Is there an association between this disorder and lung cancer?

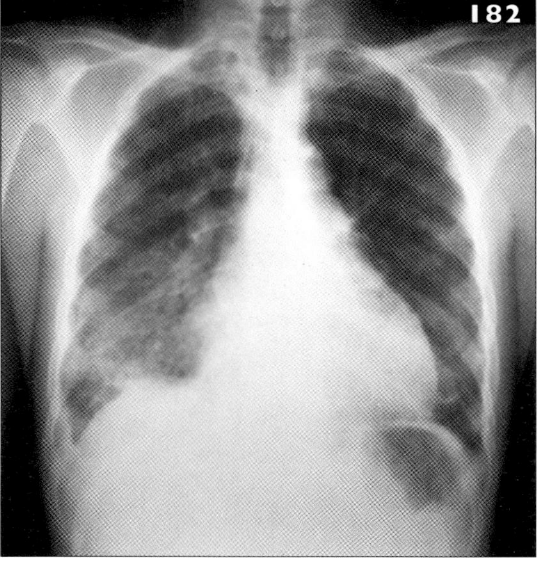

181 i. The chest radiograph (**181**) shows enlargement of the pulmonary arteries, suggesting pulmonary hypertension.

ii. The combination of pulmonary hypertension and hepatic failure should suggest the diagnosis of schistosomiasis when the patients originate from areas in which this infection occurs. Schistosomiasis is caused by one of the blood flukes, *Schistosoma mansoni*, *S. japonica* or *S. haematobia*, which are endemic to tropical areas with an appropriate intermediate host population of freshwater snails. Free-swimming cercariae penetrate human skin, then become schistosomulae which migrate through the lungs to mature in specific mesenteric venous plexuses. Pulmonary manifestations including cough, wheezing, and infiltrates can accompany the systemic symptoms of 'Katayama Fever' during the migration of schistosomulae through the lungs in acute schistosomiasis. Eggs produced by the mature flukes are carried downstream from the mesentery and lodge in the liver. A massive and inappropriate granulomatous inflammatory response to the schistosomal eggs then results in tissue injury and fibrosis. The liver eventually becomes cirrhotic and portosystemic collateral channels permit embolic eggs to reach the lungs where a similar inflammatory response ensues. The end result is pulmonary hypertension and cor pulmonale.

iii. The diagnosis of schistosomiasis is based on the identification of eggs in the stool or urine of patients having a compatible clinical presentation and a history of travel or residence in an endemic area (parts of South America, the Caribbean, Africa, and the Middle and Far East).

iv. Treatment with praziquantel is effective in preventing further egg production but may not improve established lesions.

182 i. Cough and dyspnoea on exertion are the most common presenting symptoms in patients with IPF. Up to one-half of patients have systemic complaints such as fever, fatigue, weight loss, myalgias or arthralgias. Fine 'Velcro' crackles may be heard late in inspiration, particularly at the bases. Early in the disease auscultation of the chest may be normal. Clubbing of the fingers and toes may occur. Cyanosis and signs of pulmonary hypertension, with or without cor pulmonale, are late findings.

Pulmonary function abnormalities include a reduction in lung volumes, often with the vital capacity being reduced out of proportion to the other volumes. Spirometry may be normal in the early stages. Single breath diffusing capacity for carbon monoxide (DL_{CO}) is reduced. In the later stages of the disease, arterial blood gas tension may show resting hypoxaemia. In a young female, an underlying connective tissue disease such as SLE or rheumatoid arthritis should be suspected.

ii. There is an increased incidence of lung cancer in patients with idiopathic pulmonary fibrosis. This increase in thought to result from the known association between scarring in the pulmonary parenchyma and the development of pulmonary neoplasm. All cell types of lung cancer can occur.

183 The chest radiographs 183a and 183b and barium swallow 183c belong to 68-year-old female.

i. What lesion is demonstrated?

ii. Of which symptoms would the patient be likely to complain?

iii. Which form of management is likely to be advised and why would it be recommended?

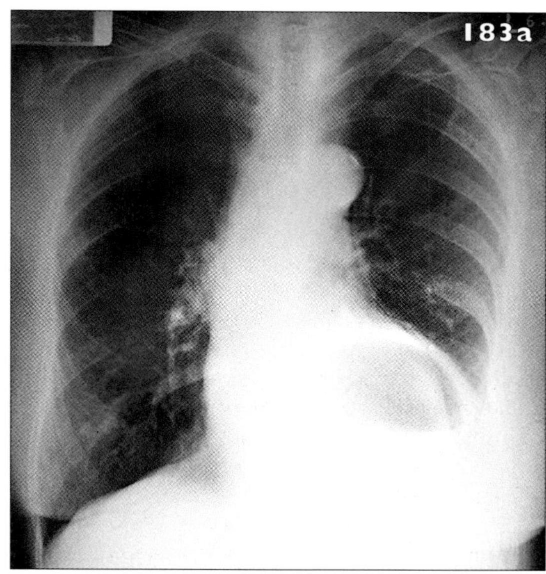

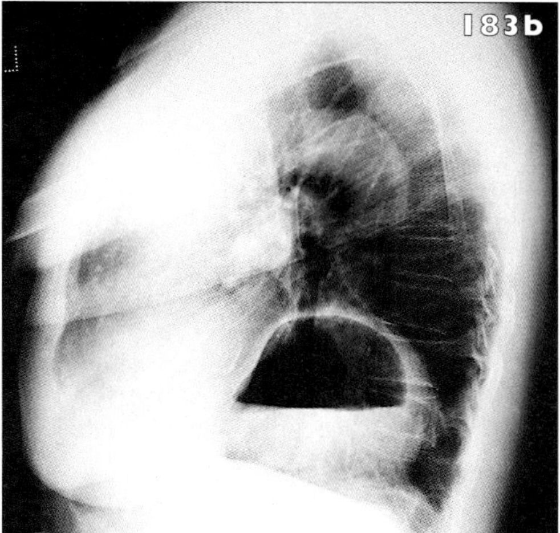

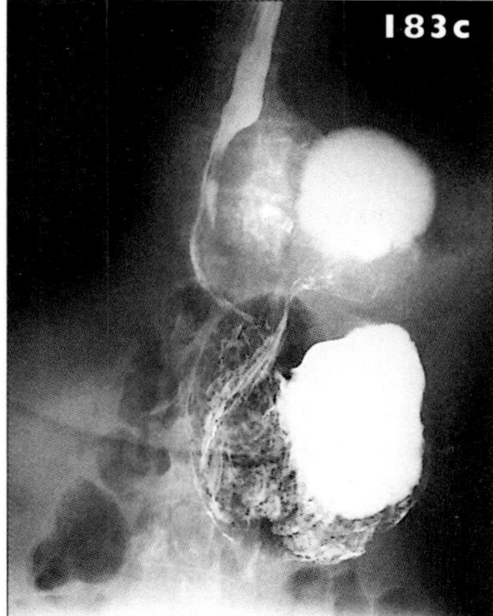

184 What are the therapeutic options for obstructive sleep apnoea (OSA)?

183 **i.** A 'rolling' hiatus hernia. In this condition the herniated stomach protrudes into the chest through the hiatus beside the lower oesophagus. The oesophagogastric junction is usually normally located.

ii. These patients may be remarkably symptom-free and the condition may be spotted as an incidental finding. Moderate dysphagia and fullness with meals are, however, common and may worsen as a meal progresses due to distension of the intrathoracic stomach. Acid reflux is not a feature because the oesophagogastric junction is usually competent and because the intrathoracic stomach further prevents reflux by pressing on the lower oesophagus.

iii. Surgical management is usually advised. This is the only effective way to manage dysphagia due to this condition and if the hernia is not reduced there is a risk of ulceration and perforation or even strangulation of the herniated stomach.

Reduction of the hernia may be accomplished via a low left lateral thoracotomy or a laparotomy. Advantages of a thoracic approach include better access to the oesophagogastric junction and hernia sac. An abdominal approach may be helpful in the event that concurrent abdominal surgery is required but offers poorer access to divide the adhesions, which are frequently present in the hernial sac.

184 Simple advice for patients with mild to moderate OSA includes sleeping on their side, no alcohol after 6:00 p.m., no sedatives, lose weight, stop smoking and keep the nose as clear as possible.

The medical treatment of choice is nasal continuous positive airway pressure (nasal CPAP) breathing. This is successful in patients with severe symptoms who gain considerable and rapid relief and improvement in well-being.

Surgical treatments include:

- Tonsillectomy and adenoidectomy, especially in children with enlarged tonsils and adenoids which can cause OSA.
- Uvulopalatopharyngoplasty – (see 88).
- Nasal surgery – generally not useful except in a few who benefit from anterior nasal reconstruction, septal straightening and polyp removal.
- Maxilla and/or mandibular advancement, a major operation bringing forward the mandible and the maxilla to preserve teeth alignment. This is only appropriate if there is a considerable degree of retrognathia with a very narrow retroglossal space and if the patient is unable to tolerate nasal CPAP.
- Tracheostomy. This was used before the availability of nasal CPAP. The tracheostomy is kept closed during the day and open at night.
- Weight loss by gastric surgery – gastroplasty has become popular in some centres.

185 The building shown (**185**) is located at the home of a 52-year-old man who presents with recurrent episodes of dyspnoea and fever. His symptoms worsen after he works in this building, especially in early spring.
i. What is the most likely diagnosis that would account for this patient's complaints?
ii. List two other antigens which can produce syndromes similar to the one described.
iii. What are the characteristic radiological manifestations of this disorder?

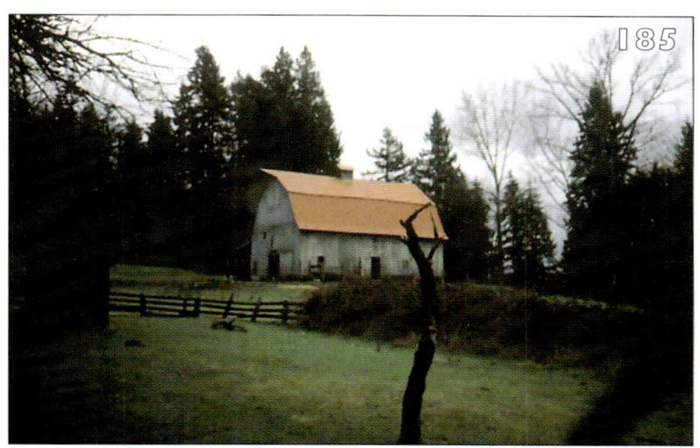

186 Shown (**186**) are pneumococci growing on a blood agar plate with a zone of inhibition around an optochen disc. This came from a sputum sample from a patient with community-acquired pneumonia.
i. What is the treatment of choice?
ii. Why may this no longer be the treatment of choice in 10 years' time?

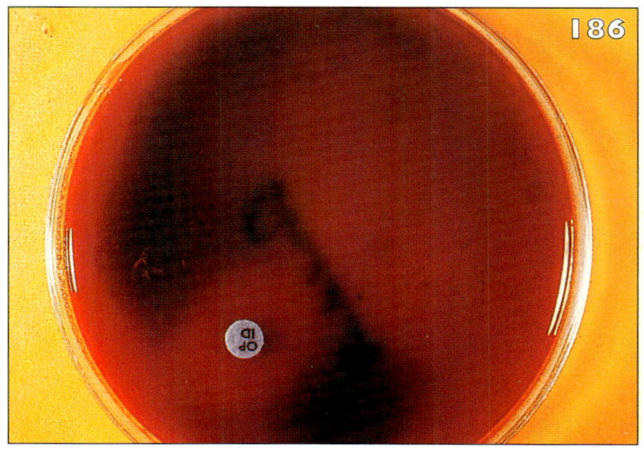

185 i. The presenting complaints are most consistent with farmer's lung, a specific syndrome which is a manifestation of hypersensitivity pneumonitis or extrinsic allergic alveolitis. The disease generally occurs after exposure to mouldy hay and is most frequently seen during the early spring or late winter months – the times of the year when previously harvested hay that has been left undisturbed for prolonged periods is used for feeding cattle. Farmer's lung results from sensitization to thermophilic bacteria, including *Thermoactinomyces volgaris* and *Micropolysporia faeni*.

ii. Other organic antigens known to cause extrinsic allergic alveolitis include avian proteins (e.g. bird fancier's lung, especially pigeons and budgerigars), rat urine (e.g. laboratory worker's lung), *Penicillum caseii* (e.g. cheese worker's lung) and *T. sacchari* (e.g. bagassosis in sugar cane workers).

iii. Early in the disease the chest radiograph may be normal. As the condition progresses findings may include ground glass opacities, reticulonodular infiltrates and diffuse interstitial fibrosis that may evolve into a honeycomb pattern with loss of lung volume. This would only occur in the setting of prolonged exposure; therefore, once the condition is diagnosed, removal of the subject from the offending allergen is the main objective. Face masks should also be worn at times when exposure to airborne fungal spores from mouldy crops may occur. Steroids may have a place in treatment; however, if the exposure has been very prolonged and insidious (e.g. with budgerigars) the disease may have caused extensive pulmonary damage. Steroids and removing the birds seem to produce scant improvement.

186 i. A penicillin is the treatment of choice. Benzylpenicillin remains the best of the penicillins, but for the patient requiring oral therapy an amino-penicillin such as amoxicillin is probably as good. For the patient allergic to penicillin a macrolide is the best alternative. Oral cephalosporins, sulphonamides, tetracyclines and quinolones are generally less effective.

ii. Pneumococcal penicillin resistance was first reported in Australia in 1967 and is now documented to be a worldwide problem. The frequency of penicillin resistance in pneumococci varies geographically, being particularly common in South Africa, Spain and Eastern Europe and rare in the United Kingdom and Scandinavia. However, every country which has looked for the problem has found it and shown a progressive rise in the frequency of pneumococcal penicillin resistance. For CNS infections this means that penicillins are no longer the treatment of choice. However, since the resistance is a graded phenomenon for pulmonary infections where the pneumococcus is of intermediate resistance, penicillins in high doses still appear to work. Nonetheless, alternative antibiotics are probably first-line treatment for high-level penicillin resistance which, fortunately, currently is rare. Pneumococcal resistance to other commonly used antibiotics such as cephalosporins and macrolides is also rising.

187 These two patients were referred for diagnostic mediastinal biopsy. Dyspnoea was a feature of patient A (**187a, 187b**), and hoarseness of patient B (**187c, 187d**).

i. What radiological features are present in these cases and why do they have the symptoms described?

ii. What method of access might be appropriate to obtain the diagnostic samples?

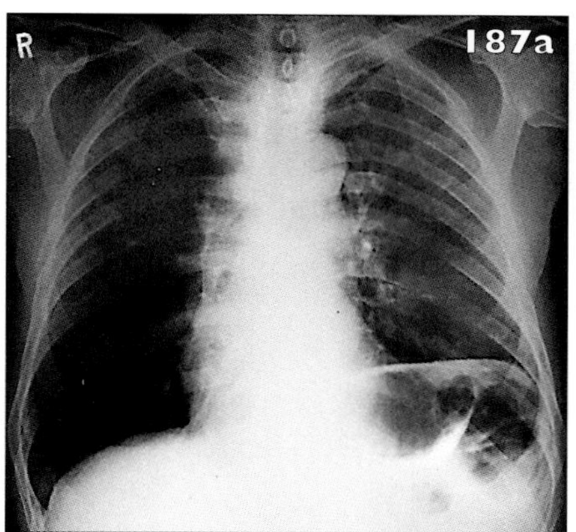

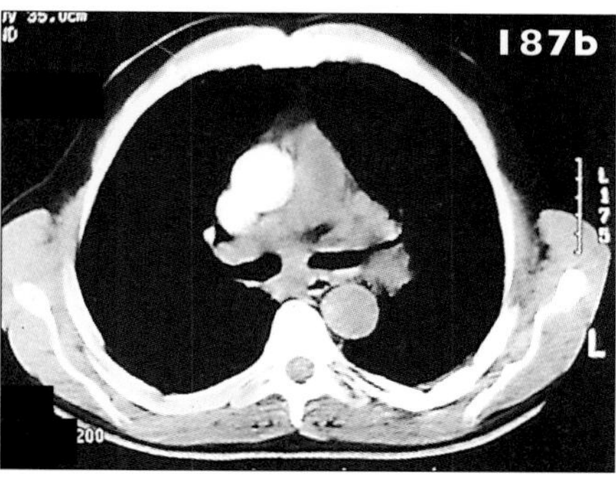

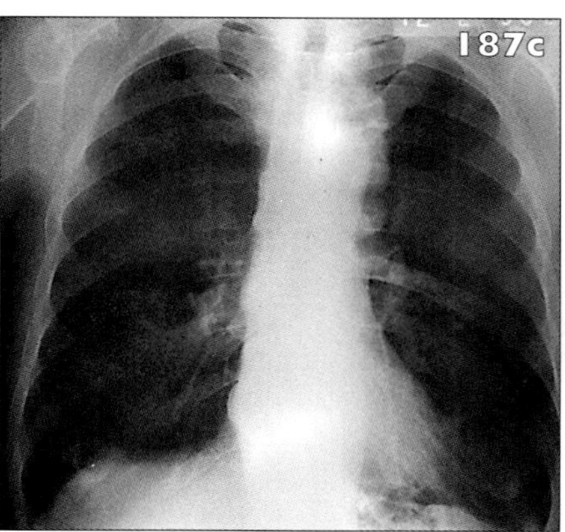

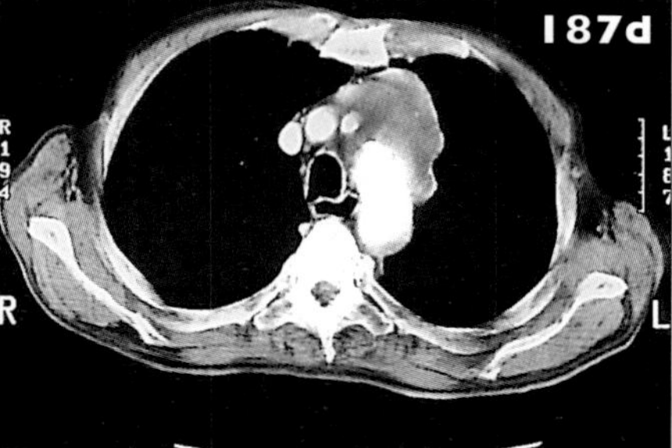

188 A patient with stage II sarcoidosis has moderate exertional dyspnoea, cough and lethargy.

i. What lung function tests would you order and what would you find?

187 i. Patient A (**187a, 187b**) has a large irregular mass in the visceral compartment extending from hilar level to the thoracic inlet. The left diaphragm is elevated due to phrenic nerve involvement. The mass is due to gross lymphadenopathy which is clearly visible on the CT cut in the subcarinal and subaortic areas. This patient clearly has either advanced lymphoma or disseminated bronchial carcinoma.

Patient B (**187c, 187d**) has a mass in the upper part of the visceral compartment which is associated with tracheal deviation to the right. The mass has caused only partial obliteration of the aortic knuckle, suggesting that it must lie quite anteriorly. This is confirmed on the CT cut where the mass can be seen applied to the anterior end of the aortic arch. Vascular involvement would preclude excision and the hoarseness of voice, due to involvement of the left recurrent laryngeal nerve, suggests significant disease in the subaortic and medial aortic areas.
ii. Biopsy in patient A would be best undertaken by mediastinoscopy in the first instance as there is significant central lymphadenopathy. (Adenocarcinoma was diagnosed in subcarinal and anterior carinal node samples.)

Patient B has disease which might be difficult to access at mediastinoscopy but which could be sampled via a left anterior mediastinotomy or by a video-assisted thorascopic surgery (VATS) approach. (Small-cell carcinoma was present in the para-aortic mass).

188 i. Although sarcoidosis characteristically causes a restrictive ventilatory defect with reduced lung volumes, lung compliance and gas exchange, it may also cause significant airflow obstruction both of small and large airways. Occasionally it causes upper airways obstruction and laryngeal involvement and rarely sleep apnoea. Flow volume loops, full lung volumes and diffusing capacity would help in assessment and follow-up. A mixed obstructive/restrictive ventilatory defect or even a purely obstructive defect may be found. Even in stage I disease significant lung function abnormalities including reduced diffusing capacity commonly occur. Although the respiratory muscles may be affected it rarely causes any functional problem. Exercise testing (cycle ergometry) may be useful in selected patients and can also detect hitherto unsuspected cardiac involvement. A fibreoptic bronchoscopy is advisable for suspected endobronchial sarcoid especially in the presence of obstructive spirometry, and to exclude other causes of cough. Stage III and IV disease is more likely to be associated with more severe reductions in diffusing capacity, which may also be due to damage to the pulmonary vasculature. Usually with corticosteroid treatment lung volumes improve sooner than carbon monoxide uptake.

189 i. How would you manage a young man presenting with this chest radiograph (**189**) for the first time?
ii. What is the risk of recurrence?
iii. How would you manage this?

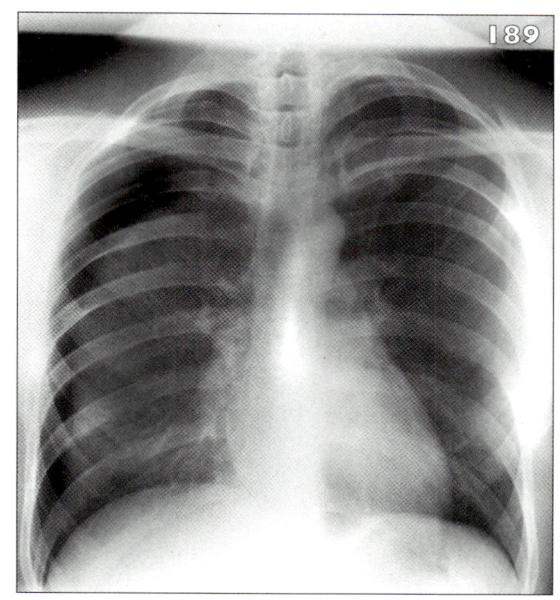

190 i. What abnormality is present on the flow–volume curve in **190**?
ii. Explain the pathophysiology.
iii. What are possible causes?

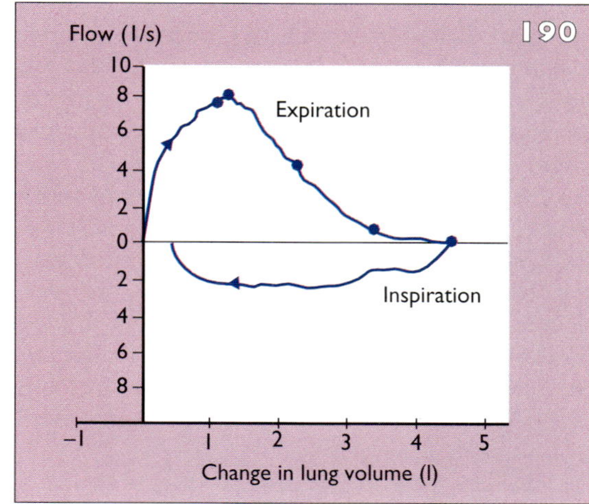

189 i. The majority of spontaneous pneumothoraces occur as a result of rupture of subpleural apical blebs in otherwise fit and healthy individuals. Rarely there is an underlying inflammatory or degenerative disease process such as TB, scleroderma or interstitial pulmonary fibrosis that requires attention. If the rupture of a small bleb results in a small pneumothorax (<20%) and the patient is asymptomatic then often nothing needs to be done other than advising the patient to reduce activities. In larger pneumothoraces where the patient is breathless, the pneumothorax should be aspirated via a small cannula attached to a 50 ml syringe via a 3-way tap, introduced into the second anterior intercostal space. A volume of air up to 2.5 l can be aspirated, but the procedure should be stopped earlier if lung is blocking the needle, or no more air is coming out with ease. A chest radiograph taken 1 h later will show if the procedure has been successful. If the lung has not re-expanded then intercostal tube drainage should be undertaken. Most patients will have their lung re-expanded rapidly and will leave hospital within 5 days. If there is a persistent air leak after this time surgery should be considered.
ii. The risk of recurrence after a first, conservatively treated pneumothorax is in the order of 30–40%.
iii. A second pneumothorax should lead to consideration of surgery. The operation of choice is a pleurectomy, giving a 95–98% chance of no further recurrence. Pleural abrasion is an acceptable alternative.

190 i. The flow–volume loop demonstrates an extrathoracic obstruction, with greatly reduced inspiratory flow with preserved expiratory flow.
ii. As the expiratory flow curve is normal (i.e. airway calibre must be normal) and the inspiratory loop is grossly reduced (i.e. the airway must be narrowed), the airflow obstruction must be variable, and worse during inspiration. Normally, during inspiration, the intrathoracic negative pressure pulls the intrathoracic airways open – this is not happening here and clearly suggests that the obstruction causing airway narrowing is in the upper airways outside the thoracic cage, i.e. an extrathoracic variable upper airway obstruction.

Conversely, if the obstruction was in the thorax, expiration would be abnormal, but it is preserved in an extrathoracic obstruction as this does not affect expiratory flow as much as it affects inspiratory flows. In the case shown here during forced inhalation, the pressure inside the upper airway decreases below atmospheric pressure and, unless stability is maintained by the pharyngeal muscles and other supporting structures, the cross-sectional area of the upper airway will decrease, truncating the inspiratory curve.
iii. Variable extrathoracic upper airway obstruction can be caused by tumour, fat deposits, pharyngeal muscle weakness, vocal cord paralysis or enlarged lymph nodes.

191 These three radiographs
(191a–c) were all taken within 24
hours in a patient admitted to the
ITU and ventilated for an aspiration
pneumonia. He had made
reasonable progress over the
subsequent 5 days but then suddenly
deteriorated following
physiotherapy with oxygen
saturations falling to 70% on FiO_2:
0.65. A cuff leak was detected and
an emergency change of
endotracheal (ET) tube was
performed just before the first chest
radiograph was taken.
i. Describe the appearances on the
chest radiographs and explain the
sequence of events.
ii. What are the other common
causes of an acute fall in oxygen
saturation (SaO_2) in a ventilated
patient?

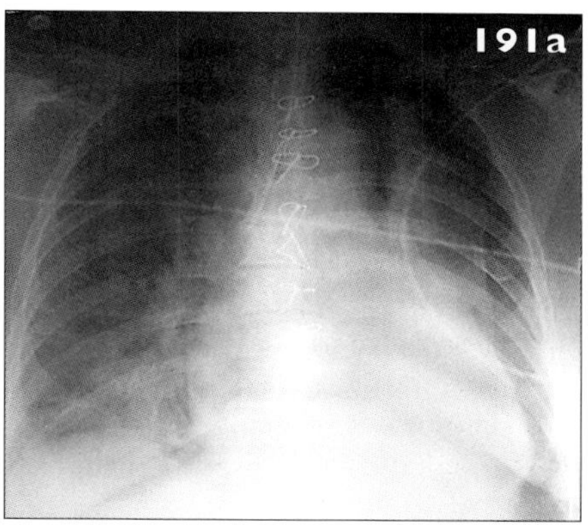

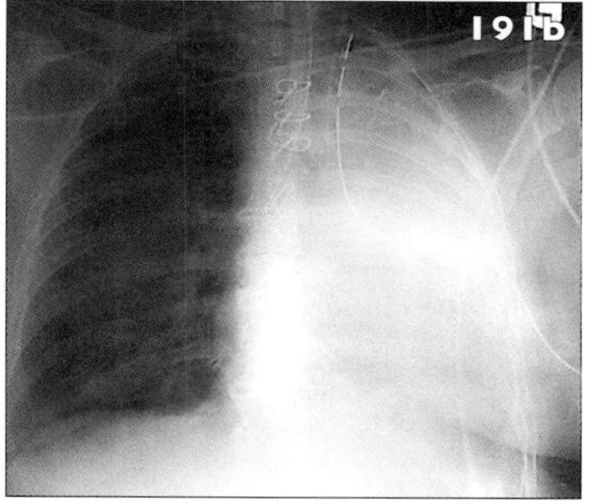

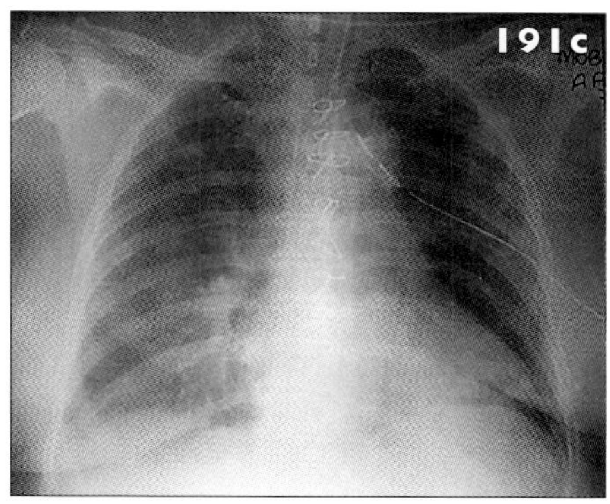

192 i. Would the management of asthma in a pregnant patient differ from
usual asthma treatment?
ii. How would pregnancy be affected by asthma?
iii. What is the effect of pregnancy on asthma?

191 The first chest radiograph (**191a**) shows a left pneumothorax and an ET tube that is too long and passed into the right main bronchus. The second radiograph (**191b**) shows the appearance after insertion of a chest drain and a complete 'whiteout' on the left side. The mediastinum is shifted to the left, indicating complete collapse of the left lung rather than a left haemothorax. The patient had been producing copious secretions and bronchoscopy revealed thick inspissated mucopurulent secretions occluding the left main bronchus and segmental bronchi. The third chest radiograph (**191c**) is taken after extensive bronchial toilet.

The sequence of events was almost certainly that physiotherapy with 'bagging' released some thick secretions that were not aspirated with routine suctioning and also led to the left pneumothorax. The emergency change of ET tube resulted in intubation of the right main bronchus.

Other causes of acute falls in oxygen saturation in ventilated patients include:
- Pulmonary oedema.
- Pulmonary embolus.
- Patient 'fighting' the ventilator – this may be due to discomfort and anxiety alone or may be precipitated by and exacerbate any of the other causes.
- Technical problems – accidental changes in ventilator settings, e.g. FiO_2, disconnection: accidental or suctioning, particularly in patients dependent on high levels of positive end-expiratory pressure (PEEP) and prolonged I:E ratios.
- Changes in posture.
- Increase in oxygen consumption: pain, anxiety, shivering/rigors, increased temperature, sepsis, drugs.

192 **i.** No, although there should be increased vigilance of asthma control particularly close to the time of delivery. Delivery is usually uncomplicated if the control is good. As with all asthmatics, inhaled therapy is preferred. No increased teratogenesis has been reported when mothers receive beta-agonists, inhaled steroids, sodium cromoglycate or theophylline. When systemic steroids are used neonatal hypoadrenalism is very rare.

ii. A prospective study of 504 pregnant asthmatic women showed that of 177 patients not initially treated with inhaled corticosteroids, 17% had an acute attack in contrast to 4% of the 257 patients who had been on inhaled anti-inflammatory treatment from the start of the pregnancy. No differences were observed between the two groups as to length of gestation, length of third stage of labour, or amount of haemorrhage after delivery. Neither were any differences observed between these groups with regard to relative birth weight, incidence of malformations, hypoglycaemia or need for phototherapy for jaundice in the neonatal period. In an earlier smaller prospective study of 198 pregnant women, there was a small increase in pre-eclampsia and a higher incidence of caesarean section in asthmatic patients compared with non-asthmatics.

iii. There is no specific effect. In about 40–50 % of women, asthma remains unchanged, in 25% it improves, and in another 25% it deteriorates.

193 This 22-year-old woman presented with non-specific malaise and an irritating cough for which her GP arranged a chest radiograph (**193a, 193b**), and a CT scan was then performed (**193c**).
i. What abnormalities are present?
ii. What diagnoses are possible?
iii. How might a diagnosis be achieved?

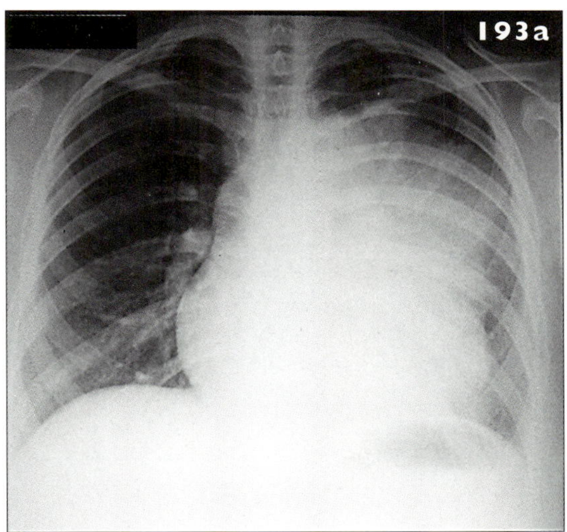

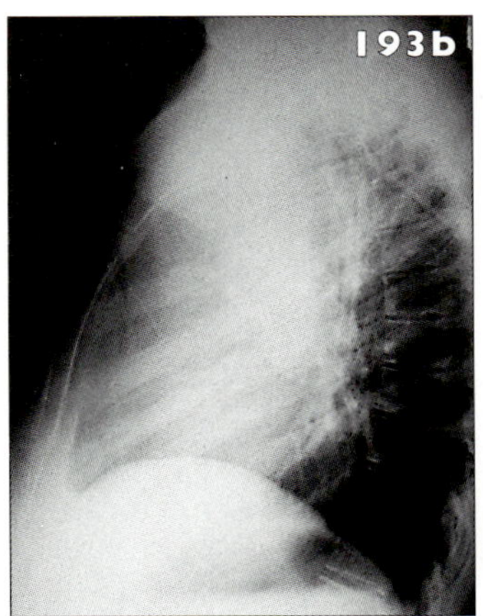

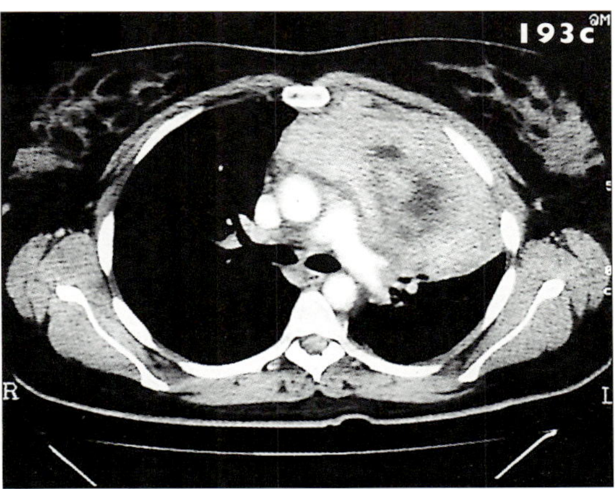

194 i. Explain the difference between occupational sensitizers and irritants as they relate to the development of asthma.
ii. Are there legal implications for the difference?

193 i. There is a huge smooth mediastinal mass located in the anterior compartment. Note that the trachea is not deviated laterally despite the left-sided preponderance of the mass suggesting an anterior origin from the plain chest film. On the CT (**193c**) there is marked posterior displacement of the visceral structures. Airway obstruction or even superior vena caval compression may occur.

ii. These appearances could be present with a variety of rapidly growing malignancies but in a female of this age group a lymphoma would be a high probability. Other possibilities would include a germ cell tumour (in a male), a thymic carcinoma, a primary sarcoma and metastatic chorioncarcinoma.

In 90% of adult cases of mediastinal lymphoma, nodular sclerosing Hodgkin's is diagnosed (as in this case); 75% of Hodgkin's patients have mediastinal involvement.

iii. Approximately half of the patients with a mediastinal lymphomatous mass have nodes palpable in the neck and excisional biopsy of one of these would be the least invasive method of getting a tissue sample. If cervical nodes are not present a CT-guided core biopsy can be performed. Anterior mediastinotomy offers a good way of obtaining a larger specimen. A right- or left-sided biopsy is performed depending upon the direction of enlargement of the mass. Mediastinoscopy would be quite impossible and dangerous in a case such as this, but can be helpful in providing a diagnosis in patients with modest mediastinal lymphadenopathy.

194 i. Sensitizer-induced occupational asthma has the features of an allergic response as there is a latency period between exposure and sensitization. Once the patient is sensitized symptoms of asthma may occur on exposure to lower levels of the substance. Symptoms initially occur only in response to that substance. Sensitization is unpredictable, occurring in 5–20% of exposed individuals. Sensitization is permanent and asthma may reappear upon re-exposure to the substance after years of non-exposure. There is specific and non-specific airway hyperresponsiveness. Patients with pre-existent asthma may become sensitized to an agent upon entering a new workplace.

Irritants produce asthma without a latent period and are associated with only non-specific airway hyperresponsiveness. Examples include diesel exhaust fumes and sulphur dioxide or perfumes. Irritants possibly contribute to the sensitization process by damaging airways and preventing adequate healing after initial early exposure to sensitizers.

ii. In the UK, to qualify for industrial injuries disablement benefit the worker must have asthma caused by an identified respiratory sensitizer, whereas for common law compensation the asthma may be of any type, either sensitizer- or irritant-induced. In this case however the individual must prove that the employer was negligent with work practices substantially worse than the norm for similar employers.

195 This HIV-positive man has a CD4+ lymphocyte count of $0.15\times10^9/l$ and presents with acute onset of fever cough and dyspnoea.
i. What are the likely causes of the chest radiograph (**195a**) abnormalities?
ii. What is the actual cause as revealed in the cytological specimen (**195b**)?
iii. How frequently would this condition present as the first AIDS-defining condition?
iv. Describe the management of this patient.

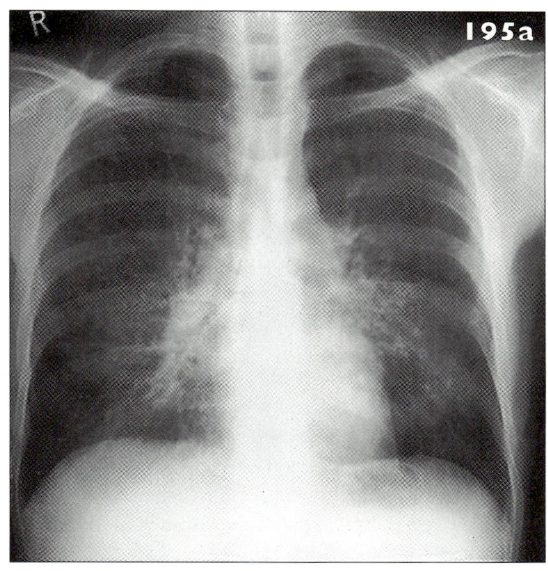

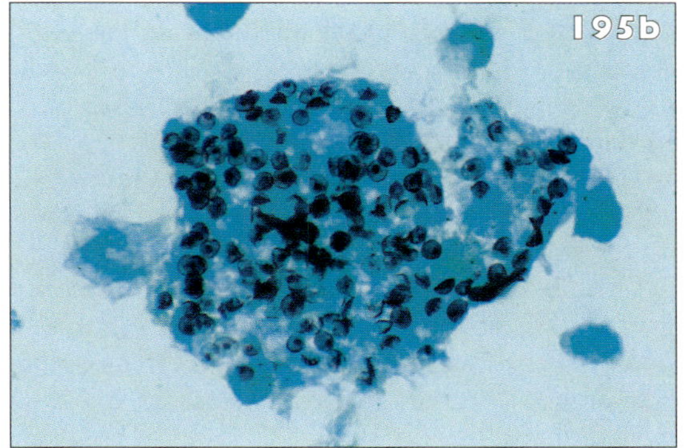

196 i. Approximately what percentage of chronic cigarette smokers develop airflow limitation?
ii. What are the benefits of smoking cessation in terms of pulmonary function?
iii. What strategies are available for aiding smoking cessation?

195 i. Bilateral interstitial shadows such as these (**195a**) are most likely to be due to *P. carinii* pneumonitis (PCP). Bacterial pneumonia, tuberculosis, histoplasmosis (in endemic areas) and pulmonary oedema due to left ventricular failure should also be considered. Infection with atypical mycobacteria, *C. neoformans* and cytomegalovirus are less likely given that the CD4 count is above $0.1 \times 10^9/l$.
ii. This bronchoalveolar lavage specimen (**195b**) has been stained with Grocott's methenamine silver and reveals numerous *P. carinii* cysts (staining black).
iii. At the start of the AIDS epidemic in the early and mid-1980s, PCP accounted for 50% of new cases of AIDS but with the more widespread use of primary prophylaxis with agents such as co-trimoxazole and nebulized pentamidine, PCP now constitutes approximately 30% of first AIDS-defining conditions.
iv. The diagnosis is usually confirmed by microscopy after silver or immunofluorescent staining of a bronchoscopic alveolar lavage specimen although a smaller proportion can be diagnosed by microscopy of sputum induced after nebulized saline. High-dose co-trimoxazole (120 mg/kg/day) is the drug of choice and is given orally or by intravenous infusion for 3 weeks. There is a high rate of reactions to this drug (rash, fever or hepatitis). Alternatives include intravenous pentamidine, clindamycin with primaquine, dapsone with trimethaprim or atovoquone. In moderate or severe cases (resting arterial PaO_2 <9.3 kPa on air) or those failing to respond quickly to antibiotics alone, a short course of high-dose glucocorticoids is beneficial. Supplemental oxygen is often required and severe cases may require ventilatory support, which is still compatible with recovery. Survivors should be given long-term prophylaxis as discussed above.

196 i. Only approximately 15% of smokers develop airflow limitation. Accordingly, other unknown factors must contribute to this problem (e.g. genetic susceptibility, other yet to be determined protease abnormalities).
ii. The rate of decline in FEV_1 in continuing smokers (~30–140 ml per year) is greater than that of ex-smokers and approaches that of non-smokers (30 ml per year). Thus, smoking cessation can reduce the rate of loss of lung function and thereby determine, to a large extent, the patient's subsequent clinical course. Clearly, much depends on the habitual activity of the subject as to when he or she presents. A manual worker may notice dyspnoea before a sedentary person. Unfortunately dyspnoea occurs with gross deterioration in lung function having already occurred in the majority of susceptible smokers.
iii. Smoking cessation clinics and hypnotherapy has been generally unsuccessful. Transdermal nicotine patches, and to a lesser extent nicotine gum seem valuable. The nicotine dose (5, 10 or 20 mg per patch) can be titrated to the patient's level of addiction. The patches should not be worn overnight. Just advising the patient not to smoke should always be offered.

197 i. What is this syndrome (**197**) most likely to be caused by?
ii. How would you make the diagnosis?
iii. How would you treat the patient?

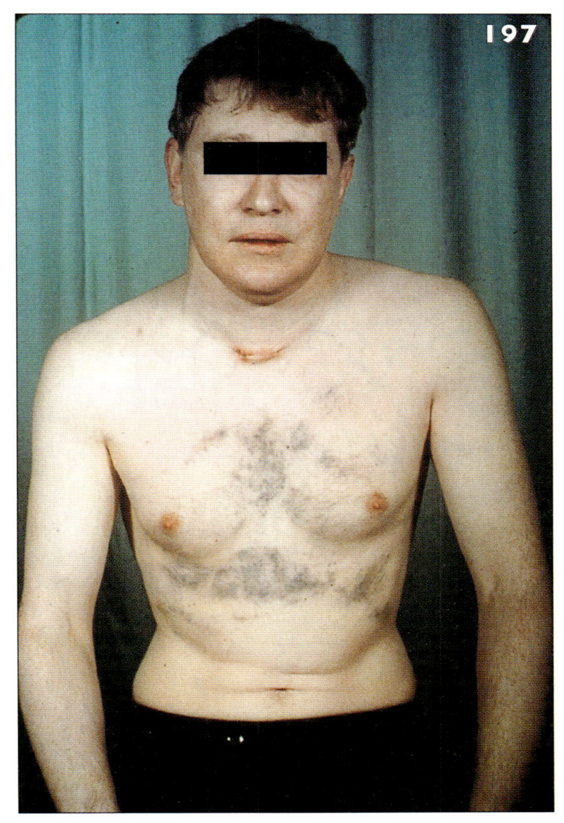

198 i. What is shown (**198**) in this asthmatic patient?
ii. What is the cause of it?
iii. Name two other local side effects of this therapy.
iv. How would you prevent this problem?

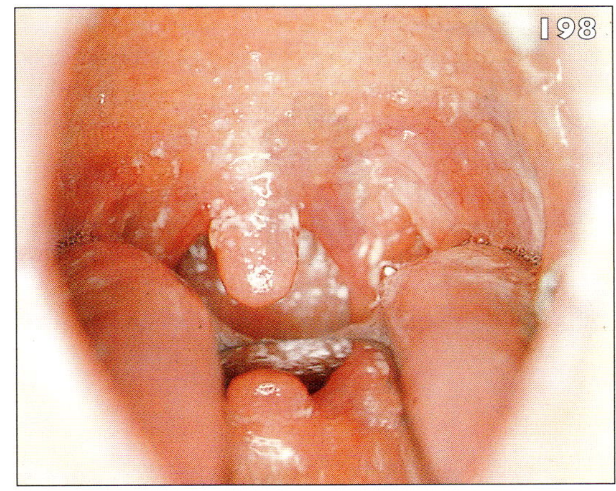

197 i. In an adult over 40 years of age, lung cancer is the most common cause of superior vena caval obstruction (SVCO) and small-cell the likeliest cell type. In a younger patient, lymphoma is the usual cause. Rarely, fibrosing conditions can affect the mediastinum and produce SVCO.

ii. In lung cancer, the diagnosis is often possible by fibre-optic bronchoscopy. A visible lesion should be brushed before biopsy to assess the likelihood of troublesome bleeding. If bronchoscopy is unhelpful, then the diagnosis will be made by mediastinoscopy, which is not a hazardous procedure as abnormal tissue will extend high into the thoracic inlet and be accessible to the surgeon. A diagnosis should always be made. There might be other sites to biopsy apart from within the chest, e.g. a supraclavicular lymph node or skin metastasis.

iii. If lymphoma, then the patient should be referred to a specialist unit for combination cytotoxic chemotherapy. If lung cancer, the differentiation from SCLC and non-small-cell lung cancer is important. If SCLC, treatment should be by combination chemotherapy and, if a complete response is obtained, then this should be consolidated by radiotherapy to the mediastinum and, if possible, the primary site.

Non-small cell lung cancer should be treated by radiotherapy. The dose will depend whether palliation or radical treatment is the intention. Cover with dexamethasone is recommended during radiotherapy.

Should the SVCO be a result of relapsed disease and it is not possible to give further radiotherapy, and the patient's general condition is reasonable, then stenting of the SVCO by a wall stent inserted via the femoral vein can provide rapid and excellent palliation.

198 i. Oral monilial infection (thrush).

ii. Inhaled corticosteroids (ICS). Oral moniliasis is the commonest side effect of this application of steroid medication. It is as common with beclomethasone and budesonide, but less frequent with fluticasone. Oropharyngeal candidiasis may occur in 5% of patients.

iii. The next most common problem is dysphonia, which may occur in up to 40% of patients and is particularly noted by teachers and singers. Laryngeal deposition of the inhaled corticosteroid causes vocal cord myopathy. It usually resolves upon cessation of inhaled steroids or changing the type of steroid. Patients with persistent dysphonia should have indirect laryngoscopy to exclude other causes.

iv. Use a spacer with metered-dose inhalers and rinse mouth after the inhaled therapy. The doses of ICS should be taken in two divided doses daily as the incidence of oral moniliasis increases with more frequent application. A course of antifungal lozenges may be necessary. Any dentures should also be treated overnight with an anti-fungal solution. This problem also occurs with dry-powder inhalers and is helped by rinsing and anti-fungal lozenges.

199 This 58-year-old man presented for a chest radiograph with an 18-month history of pain in the left upper arm and shoulder. An orthopaedic opinion a year previously advised physiotherapy. The pains continued and he developed numbness of the finger tips and difficulty performing fine movements of the hands.
i. What is the radiographic abnormality (**199a**) and what is the condition?
ii. Comment on treatment and prognosis.

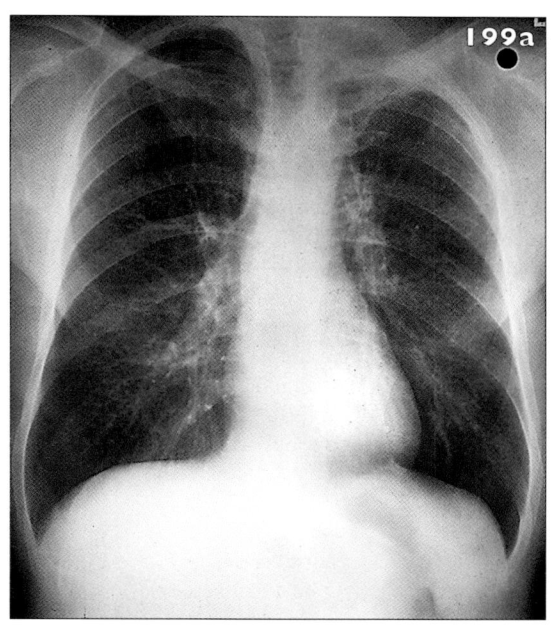

200 A confused woman of 82 years is brought to the emergency department, distressed, severely dyspnoeic and complaining of pain in the chest. A radiograph was taken (**200**). What is the diagnosis and how should the condition be managed?

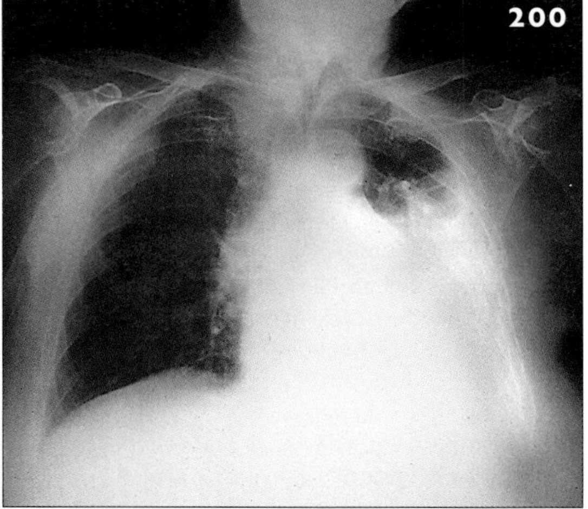

199 i. The radiograph (**199a**) shows opacification of the left apex with erosion of the posterior third of the first and second ribs. The patient has an apical, superior sulcus, tumour (Pancoast syndrome), usually an adeno or squamous cell lung cancer which grows into the brachial plexus, causing symptoms related to the T1 and C8 nerve roots. The pains are often not recognized as a brachial plexus lesion for months, often not until weakness develops in the small muscles of the hand, together with parasthesia. A CT of the tumour commonly shows extensive medial spread into a vertebral body (**199b**) as well as posterior extension through the ribs into the underlying muscle planes. This is well illustrated on the CT scan in this particular patient.

ii. The tumour is resectable if only the ribs are involved. Once it has penetrated through to the muscle layers or encroached onto a vertebral body it is no longer resectable. If unresectable, radical radiotherapy should be given. As these tumours often do not metastasize widely, pain control together with progressive loss of use of a limb is a very major problem.

200 Traumatic haemothorax. Careful examination of the radiograph (**200**) reveals the presence of rib fractures on the left side. Thorough drainage through a wide-bore intercostal drain is essential to prevent an organizing intrapleural haematoma. Blood transfusion may be necessary and pain control may present difficulties. Intercostal nerve blocks can be effective if up to four ribs are fractured. Patients who hypoventilate in this situation are at risk of stasis pneumonia. If there is a flail segment of chest wall due to rib fractures in two places, severe respiratory insufficiency may result and a period of intubation and positive-pressure ventilation may be necessary until the fractures heal and the chest wall stabilizes. Care must be taken to exclude more serious complications of chest trauma such as:

- Ruptured bronchus suggested by massive air leak from an intercostal drain and confirmed at bronchoscopy.
- Ruptured aorta causing hypotension. A CT scan or oesophageal echocardiogram will make the diagnosis here.
- Haemopericardium which causes hypotension in the setting of a raised JVP, and requires diagnostic echocardiograph.
- Ruptured oesophagus (see **94**).

201 A 52-year-old man is admitted semi-conscious with a 1-week history of dry cough, fever and headache. Two of his workmates have apparently been in hospital with pneumonia in the last month. He has signs of consolidation at the right lung base confirmed on chest radiograph and admission blood gases show a PaO_2 of 53 mmHg (7 kPa), $PaCO_2$ of 46 mmHg (6.1 kPa), pH 7.32, bicarbonate 15, base excess −2 breathing 60% oxygen.
i. What is wrong with this man?
ii. What is the relevance of the occupational history?
iii. How would you manage him?

202 This 70-year-old patient has had haemoptysis with recurrent episodes of pneumonia in the left lower lobe for 15 years. A mass (**202a, 202b**) was seen at bronchoscopy to be partially occluding the left lower lobe and was removed by laser resection. What is the likely diagnosis?

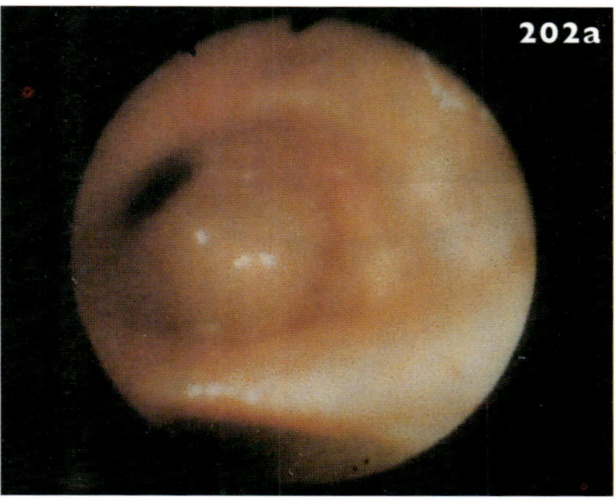

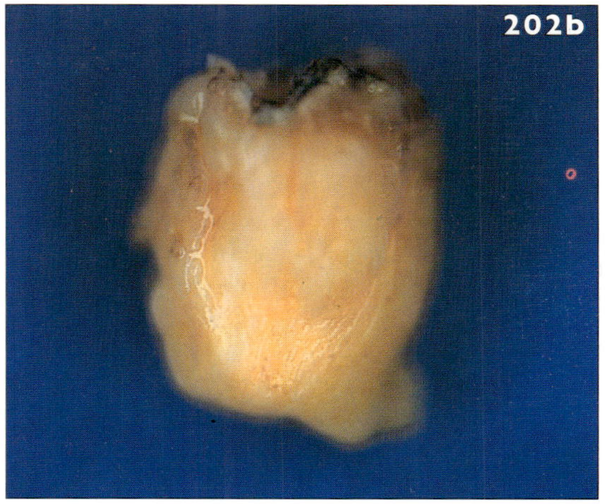

201 i. He has features of a severe community-acquired pneumonia, the presence of mental confusion, hypoxia and hypercapnia indicating that he is severely ill despite the confinement of the consolidation to his right lung.

ii. The occurrence of pneumonia in three people working in the same place suggests that they may be part of some form of outbreak. Outbreaks of pneumonia have been described with *Str. pneumoniae*, *C. psittaci*, *C. burnetti* and legionella species, the latter perhaps being top of the list unless his job involves work with animals (Q fever) or birds (psittacosis).

iii. Immediate management requires improvement in his gas exchange, fluid balance and institution of appropriate antibiotic treatment. Persisting hypoxia despite high inspired oxygen suggests that he needs additional therapy. As a first step, continuous positive airways pressure (CPAP) may be effective without running the risks of endotracheal intubation. However, this may be required together with assisted ventilation. Appropriate antibiotics would best be a combination of a second- or third-generation cephalosporin together with a macrolide to cover all of the likely common pathogens causing severe community-acquired pneumonia, mainly *Str. pneumoniae*, *H. influenzae*, *Myc. pneumoniae*, *L. pneumophila* and *Staph. aureus*. The two approaches to rapid confirmation of a diagnosis of legionnaires' disease are to examine his urine for the presence of legionella antigen and to examine a sample of a lower respiratory tract secretion, either sputum or direct lower respiratory tract aspirate, by direct fluorescent antibody staining for legionella organisms. With confirmation of a diagnosis of legionnaires' disease a macrolide remains the treatment of choice with the addition of either rifampicin or a quinolone for those who are severely ill.

202 Given the long history, this polypoid mass is likely to be a benign endobronchial tumour. The majority of these are carcinoid tumours although they can be locally invasive and metastases to hilar lymph nodes may be seen at resection. These tumours show neuroendocrine differentiation but the carcinoid syndrome is rare in bronchial carcinoids. Other benign bronchial tumours are of mesenchymal origin and include lipomas, leiomyomas and fibromas. This tumour was a mixed fibrolipoma and the laser resection line can be seen at the base of the polyp. Rigid bronchoscopy and laser were used because significant haemorrhage may occur with removal of these tumours, particularly carcinoid tumours.

Endobronchial obstruction should be suspected in cases of recurrent pneumonia, particularly when associated with haemoptysis. Inhaled foreign bodies may cause the same syndrome. Foreign bodies may not be visible on chest radiographs. Other non-malignant causes of endobronchial obstruction include amyloidosis and tracheopathia osteoplastica, a cartilaginous proliferation in the major airways. The latter may be a long-term sequel of amyloidosis. Both of these conditions may be resected using laser if the obstruction is symptomatic.

203 Shown (**203**) is the chest radiograph of a 39-year-old man with the acquired immunodeficiency syndrome who had no prior respiratory complications. He presented with symptoms of fever, headache, stiff neck and cough. The patient was born and raised in Arizona but had lived for 12 years in the Pacific Northwest.
i. What are the radiographic findings?
ii. What diseases could account for the clinical and radiological abnormalities?

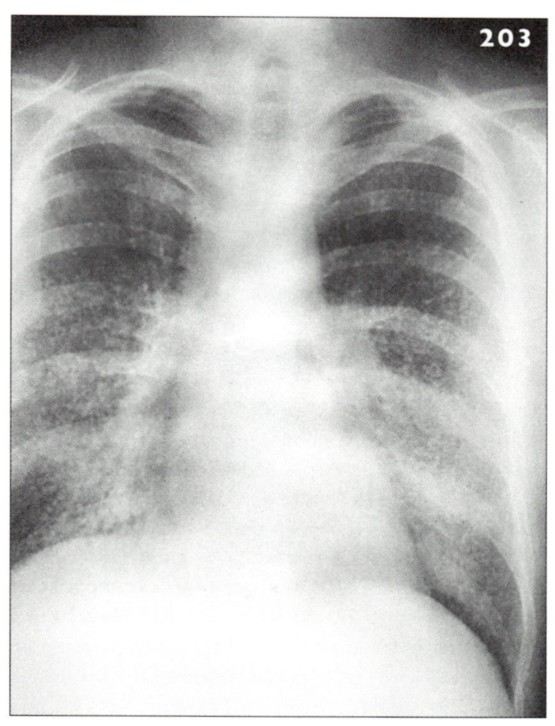

204 A previously healthy 28-year-old male complains of wheezing and dyspnoea which worsens over the working week and improves at weekends. He has been employed in a car body repair shop (**204**) for 5 years and routinely performs work shown in the accompanying figure but occasionally forgets to use his respirator. Spirometry performed at the end of a working week demonstrates reversible airflow limitation. His chest radiograph is normal.

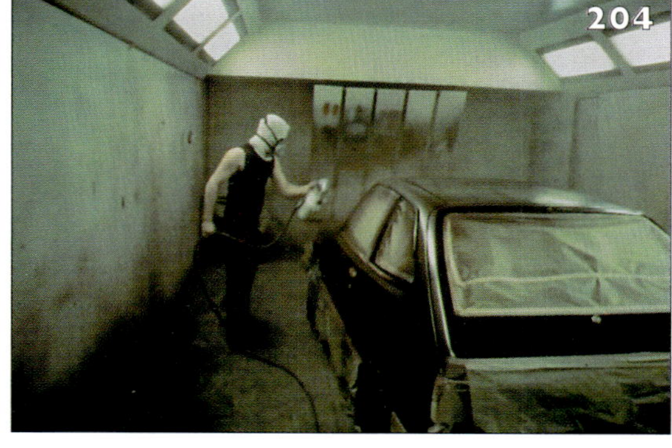

i. What is the most likely diagnosis?
ii. What is the likely offending agent?

203 i. The chest radiograph (203) shows diffuse nodular infiltrates and hilar and mediastinal adenopathy.

ii. Disseminated (miliary) tuberculosis or disseminated fungal infections could explain both the radiographic appearance and the meningeal symptoms. *P. carinii* rarely causes adenopathy. The geographic or endemic fungi, *Histoplasma capsulatum*, *Blastomyces dermatitidis*, *Paracoccidioides braziliensis* and *Coccidioides immitis* as well as the ubiquitous *C. neoformans* could all cause this presentation. *C. immitis* was especially likely based on the history of residence in an endemic area. Coccidioidomycosis is acquired by inhalation of arthrospores in the endemic area (the south-western United States and Northern Mexico). Most infected persons remain asymptomatic although they usually develop skin test reactivity. Some experience a self-limited but sometimes severe syndrome termed 'valley fever' which includes cough, fever, pleuritic chest pain, headache and arthralgias, often accompanied by a skin rash. The radiographic findings of primary coccidioidomycosis include localized infiltrates and hilar adenopathy. Healing with calcification or thin-walled cavity formation is common. Persistent primary coccidioidomycosis is the term used to continued symptoms and radiographic progression after 6 weeks. Dissemination can occur, more commonly in immunocompromised patients, pregnant women, and in dark-skinned races. The skin, bones and joints, and meninges are most commonly involved. A definitive diagnosis is made by the isolation of *C. immitis* or by the identification of characteristic spherules containing endospores in sputum or histological specimens. Serial serological testing can be useful for following disease activity. Primary pulmonary coccidioidomycosis usually requires no treatment. Persistent or disseminated infection should be treated with systemic antifungal therapy. Amphotericin B, fluconazole and itraconazole all have activity against but most clinicians favour amphotericin B as initial therapy. Immunocompromised patients require chronic suppressive itraconazole therapy.

204 i. Occupational asthma. Wheezing, dyspnoea, reversible airflow limitation and the normal chest radiograph secure the diagnosis of asthma. Worsening symptoms during the working week with recovery over the weekend, or while on vacation, in a patient with known or suspected workplace exposure to a sensitizing compound strongly suggest occupational asthma.

ii. Diisocyanates are potent, low-molecular weight sensitizers that are widely used in polyurethane. Toluene diisocyanate (TDI), diphenyl methane diisocyanate (MDI), and hexamethylene diisocyanate (HDI) are the most commonly encountered and have all been linked to occupational asthma. HDI is a component of urethane paints used in automotive body repair and is the most likely cause of occupational asthma in this case.

Serial self-measurement of peak expiratory flow rates (PEFR) performed over 2 weeks at work and 2 weeks at home is often helpful with making the diagnosis. A 20% decrement in PEFR during or after work with recovery away from the workplace is diagnostic. Occasionally, specific bronchoprovocation testing with the suspected allergen or a workplace challenge may be required.

205 A 72-year-old man presented to his general practitioner with a history of hoarseness. Other than moderate hypertension, he had no other past history of note. A radiograph (**205a**) and CT (**205b**) were done.
i. What abnormality is present and what is the likely aetiology?
ii. What classification system can be applied to this abnormality?
iii. Why is the patient hoarse?
iv. How would this condition be managed and what risks should be discussed with the patient?

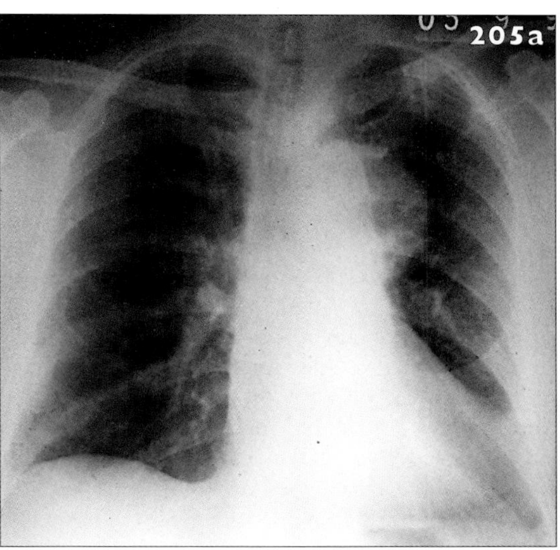

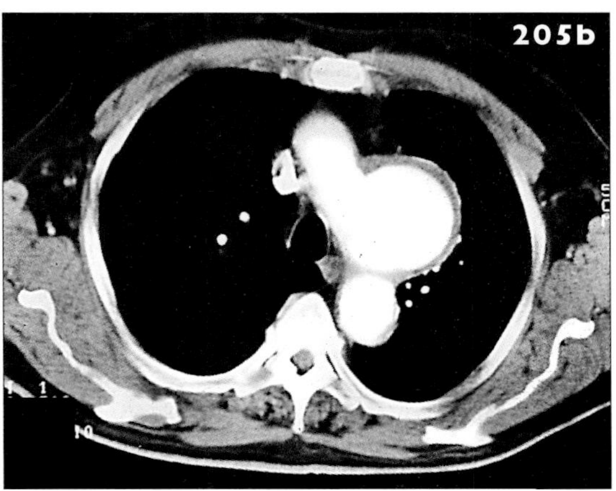

206 A CF patient may wait a year following listing for organ transplantation. Which are the clinical areas that most need close medical attention to ensure fitness for eventual transplantation?

205 i. This patient has a large aneurysm of the aortic arch. The most likely aetiology is hypertension, but syphilis serological testing would be appropriate. If it had been located at the junction of the arch and descending aorta a post-traumatic origin would have been a possibility.

ii. Aortic aneurysms may be classified in several ways. A 'true' aneurysm is contained within all the layers of the aortic wall, although these may be greatly thinned and it is common for the aneurysm to be lined with old and new thrombus. Depending on the appearance of the aneurysm, it may be described as 'saccular', as in this case, or 'fusiform' if the dilatation is more cylindrical.

If the aneurysm is formed from a localized hole in the aortic wall connecting with a cavity lined only by thrombus, it is described as a 'false' aneurysm.

An aortic dissection is often labelled as a 'dissecting aneurysm'. This condition is characterized by the entry of blood into the layers of the aortic wall through a split in the intima with prograde and/or retrograde extension of this process along a variable length of the aorta.

iii. The left recurrent laryngeal nerve has been stretched by the aneurysm.

iv. Hypertension should be controlled and the aneurysm size monitored. If it is static a conservative approach may be appropriate in someone of moderate general health or advanced age in view of the operative risk. Expansion would dictate surgical excision, probably with replacement of the aortic arch under hypothermic circulatory arrest. The patient should be warned of the magnitude of operative risk (>10% mortality) and advised specifically of the additional risk of perioperative cerebral damage.

206 Clinical areas include:
- Pulmonary sepsis must be controlled. Intensive treatment may require continuous antibiotics. Physiotherapy may need to be increased. New treatments such as DNase, which decrease sputum viscosity, may help some potential transplant recipients by improving physiotherapy and decreasing breathlessness.
- Nutrition and body weight must be maintained. Patients awaiting transplantation are hypercatabolic and have a poor appetite. Body weight can be maintained either with nasogastric feeding or gastrosotomy feeding. A gastrosotomy is the best-tolerated option. This can be used to provide overnight feeding and may also be used following transplantation.
- Respiratory failure with carbon dioxide retention can be treated with nocturnal nasal ventilation. This allows provision of safe nocturnal oxygen supplementation, rests respiratory muscles and allows mobility during the day.
- Mobility must be maintained. This can be achieved with gentle exercise. If the patient is very breathless, supplemental oxygen can be used.

All CF patients listed for transplantation should receive their continuing care in an **accredited CF centre** due to the requirement for multidisciplinary care.

207 The drug sensitivities of *Mycobacterium tuberculosis* isolated from sputum in a 45-year-old TB patient are shown in the Table.
i. What are the predisposing factors to this situation?

Drug	Sensitivity
Isoniazid (H)	Resistant
Rifampicin (R)	Resistant
Ethambutol (E)	Sensitive
Pyrazinamide (Z)	Sensitive
Streptomycin (S)	Sensitive

208 The tracing in **208** is from a young woman who complains of excessive daytime somnolence. Her bed partner also notes that she snores.
i. What is the name of her breathing-related sleep disturbance and what are the clinical and polysomnographic features of this disorder?
ii. How is this diagnosis confirmed?
iii. What is the treatment of this disorder?

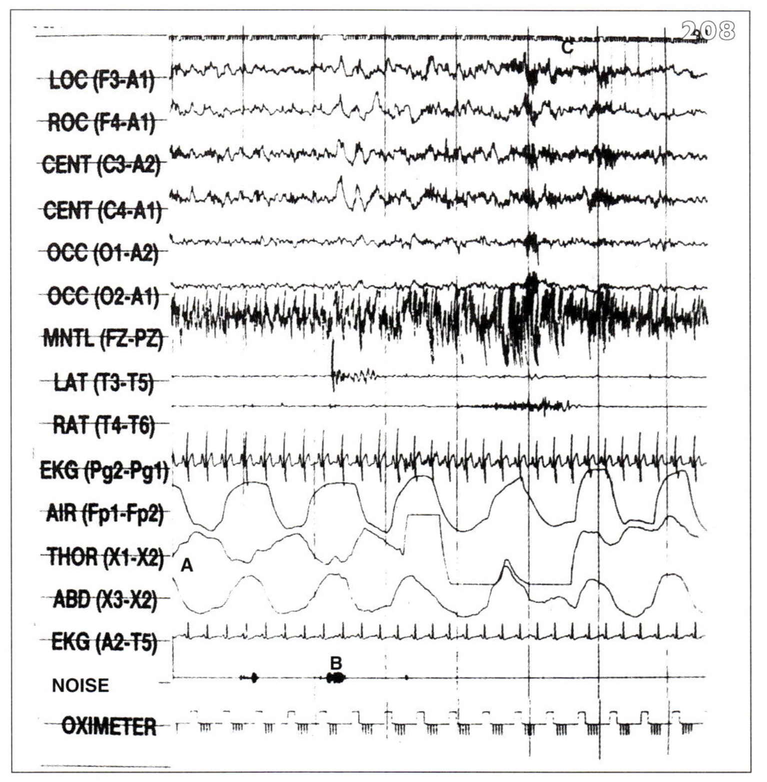

207 i. Drug-resistant TB is usually seen in patients who have had prior treatment for TB which was not completed or included inappropriate drug doses or combinations. Poor compliance is the major factor particularly in the inner cities, and is common in the vagrants, alcoholics and underprivileged subjects who contract the disease. The normal length of treatment of tuberculosis is 6 months and multiple drugs are used because *M. tuberculosis* infections normally include a small percentage of resistant bacteria which may be 'selected' if single drugs are used. Also, different drugs affect organisms at different sites where they may be growing (intracellular or extracellular). The most active anti-tuberculous drugs are isoniazid and rifampicin, as both are bactericidal and in combination prevent the development of bacterial resistance. Primary resistance (in patients not previously treated) also occurs and is most common in patients from areas where drug-resistant TB is most common (Africa, Asia, Latin America),
ii. These patients need close supervision and directly observed therapy. Where H resistance alone occurs, R, S, P and E should be given for 2 months followed by 7 months of ER. Where there is resistance to both H and R, as in this case, the regimen should include at least three drugs to which there is known sensitivity, and preferably drugs the patient has not received previously. Treatment should continue for 9 months to 2 years after sputum cultures are negative. To prevent the further development of resistance, new drugs should be added in combinations of two or three. Therefore, second line drugs are needed and include ethionamide, cycloserine, PAS, amikacin, ciprofloxacin and clofazimine. However, all of these drugs are associated with a higher incidence of side effects and are less effective than the first-line agents.

208 i. This patient has upper airway resistance syndrome. These patients present with excessive daytime somnolence. In the majority a history of snoring can be elicited. They are generally non-obese and have characteristic anatomical features including: a triangular face, a steep mandibular plane, a highly arched palate, and a class II malocclusion or a retroposition of the mandible. Standard polysomnograms show repetitive, transient alpha EEG arousals following increases in snoring. No significant change in oxygen saturation is seen and the respiratory disturbance index is low (<5). On this tracing paradoxical thoracic and abdominal movements (A) and snoring (B) are seen during the event, which is terminated by an arousal (C).
ii. Oesophageal pressure monitoring during polygraphic monitoring is helpful in demonstrating increases in respiratory effort that occur with each breath before a transient decrease in airflow which triggers arousal.
iii. A therapeutic trial of nasal CPAP. The patient should demonstrate subjective and objective evidence of improvement in daytime somnolence within 1 month.

209 Shown are the chest radiograph (**209a**) and CT scan (**209b**) of a 14-year-old boy from Alaska whose only complaint is a non-productive cough.
i. What are the radiographic abnormalities?
ii. What is the most likely diagnosis?
iii. How can this diagnosis be established?

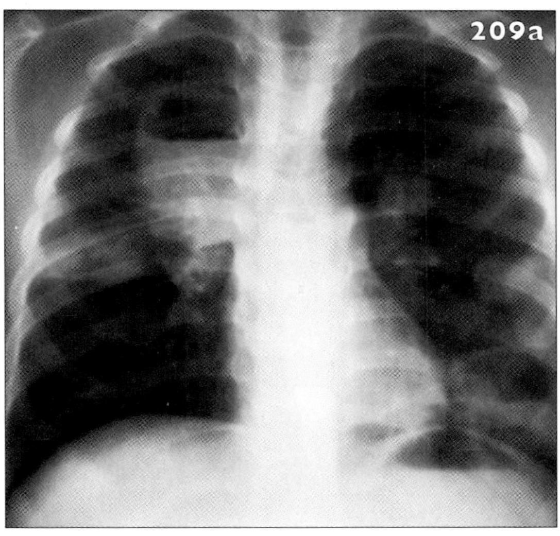

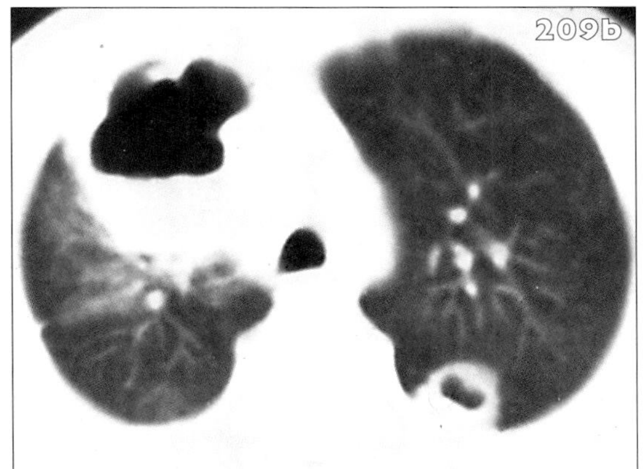

210 A pleural effusion in a 45-year-old woman was milky white. Investigations confirmed a high level of triglycerides but no cholesterol crystals. What does this imply and what are the possible causes?

211 What is the ILO classification for pneumoconiosis?

209 i. There are multiple, spherical lesions with smooth margins. The chest CT shows that most of these are moderately thin-walled cysts, many of which contain air-fluid levels.

ii. Cystic abnormalities of this size are most likely the result of Echinococcal infection. Pulmonary sequestrations may occasionally manifest in this fashion as may infected bullae or bronchogenic cysts. Sequestrations are almost always in the lower lobes and usually the left.

iii. Echinococcosis results from the ingestion of eggs of the ubiquitous carnivore tapeworms *Echinococcus granulosa* or *E. multilocularis*, prevalent in areas where dogs coexist with the natural intermediate hosts (i.e. sheep and cattle). Oncospheres released in the gut enter the portal circulation and larvae then develop in the liver, lungs or, less commonly other systemic sites. *E. granulosa* larvae form encapsulated cysts (cystic hydatid disease) which grow slowly and cause symptoms only if they rupture, become secondarily infected, or reach sufficient size to compress adjacent structures. The chest radiograph typically shows one or more homogenous masses with sharply defined margins. The 'lily pad' sign may be present if air enters the cyst. This results from collapsed cyst walls and debris floating on the surface of the fluid. Eosinophilia may be present and serological tests are usually positive. CT, and particularly MRI scanning, can reveal the cystic nature of these lesions and can identify coexistent hepatic cysts. Needle biopsy of suspected hydatid cysts should be *avoided* and treatment by intact surgical excision is desirable because spillage of cyst contents can cause anaphylaxis and may lead to larval dissemination. *E. multilocularis* cysts fail to mature and the invading scolices cause continued inflammation and tissue destruction (alveolar hydatid disease). Pulmonary involvement is focal or diffuse and treatment with systemic antihelminthic drugs is recommended (e.g. praziquantel or mebendazole).

210 Chylothorax. The presence of multiple small fat globules in the pleural fluid produces a milky white appearance. The most likely cause is accumulation of lymph due to obstruction of, or damage to, the lymphatic duct. This may be due to chest trauma or surgery of the aorta or oesophagus. Chylothorax may also be due to obstruction of the thoracic duct by lymphoma (as in this case) or other mediastinal tumours.

The onset is often acute with dyspnoea. The patient can become malnourished and immunocompromised although the effusion itself remains sterile. It has to be distinguished from an empyema, and from a chyliform or pseudochylous effusion that is often chronic and occurs in long-standing tuberculosis or rheumatoid disease. They contain high levels of lecithin or globulin complexes or cholesterol crystals.

Treatment is that of the underlying cause, though repeated aspiration may be necessary. Ligation of the thoracic duct may occasionally be necessary. Feeding with medium-chain triglyceride diets or total parenteral nutrition decreases thoracic duct flow and maintains the nutritional status. Most cases of traumatic rupture of the thoracic duct resolve in 2 weeks.

211 It is a method of grading the size of opacities on chest radiography due to pneumoconiosis, primarily for epidemiological reporting. The number of opacities correlates with the quantity of dust in the lungs. The opacities may be the dust itself or the consequent fibrosis. There is a broad division between opacities up to 1 cm (simple pneumoconiosis), and those >1 cm diameter (complicated pneumoconiosis, or progressive massive fibrosis, PMF). PMF arises on a background of simple pneumoconiosis. Profusion gives an estimate of the density of the nodules, and is determined by comparison with a set of standardized radiographs (Tables).

Each profusion category can be subdivided into three, to give a 12-point scale.

p nodules are mostly seen in coal workers' pneumoconiosis (CWP) whereas r nodules are associated with silicosis.

Lung function changes with simple CWP are usually minimal and often overshadowed by the effects of cigarette smoking, although coal dust does contribute to the development of emphysema. Radiographic changes do not progress after the miner leaves the coal face with simple CWP but they can occur with PMF. However, with silica exposure simple changes may progress despite removal from the offending agent. Those developing PMF have usually been exposed to a high dust burden. Progressive hypoxaemia usually occurs. It is important to exclude other causes of large irregular opacities such as tumours and infection.

Simple			
Nodule size	**Rounded nodules**	**Irregular nodules**	**Profusion of nodules**
<1.5 mm	p	s	0, 1, 2 or 3
1.5–3 mm	q	t	0, 1, 2 or 3
3–10 mm	r	u	0, 1, 2 or 3

Complicated	
Nodule size	**Category**
1–5 cm, or several with combined diameter up to 5 cm	A
Between A and B	B
One or more with combined area >1/3 of lung field	C

Index

Numbers refer to questions and answers, not pages.

Index